# RealRyder®
# Indoor Cycling
# Certified Instructor
# Training Manual

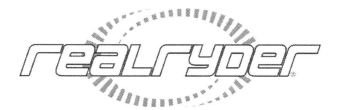

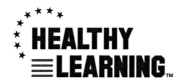

ISBN: 978-1-60679-168-4
Library of Congress Control Number: 2011923037
Cover design: Wendy Saade and Brenden Murphy
Layout design: Roger W. Rybkowski

Healthy Learning
P.O. Box 1828
Monterey, CA 93942
www.healthylearning.com

# Legal Statement

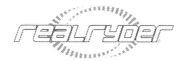

This is a manual that has been prepared by RealRyder International LLC, only for use by those instructors who are taking or who have completed the RealRyder instructor training certification. Any use of this manual by someone who has not undergone RealRyder training is strictly forbidden.

The materials contained in this manual are intended to supplement the information provided as part of the RealRyder instructor training program, and this manual is not a substitute for completing RealRyder's training, nor is it a substitute for good judgment and common sense.

Instructors and their employers are responsible for the health and safety of individuals who use RealRyder bikes in their classes, at their facilities, or otherwise in their presence or under their supervision. The information contained in this manual is not intended to create any warranties or other assurances regarding the use or safety of, or results obtained by riding, RealRyder bikes, and RealRyder International cannot and will not have any liability for injury or other harm related to the use of RealRyder bikes by instructors or by third parties.

# Contents

# RealRyder International
# Company Background

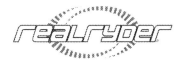

The RealRyder vision began over 15 years ago when Colin Irving, competitive cyclist and RealRyder International cofounder realized there must be a more engaging and beneficial way for cyclists to train indoors. Riding rollers or working out on a fixed stationary bike, which represented indoor training standards for decades, still left much to be desired. Inspired by a cold-weather climate and an ardent passion for cycling, Colin subsequently developed the concept of an "unstationary" bike—an indoor cycle that would better replicate and support the real bike experience. With these references in mind, Colin started thinking and sketching. His goal was to develop an indoor training tool for cyclists that would encourage and reward good form, proper pedal stroke, and appropriate position on the bike, given that these were essential skills that only rollers, real time out on the road or track could develop.

In 2005, Colin met health/wellness industry expert Sean Harrington, whose efforts in the field include work on the Heart Mate stationary bike and helping establish a successful fitness club-chain operation that featured Nautilus® equipment. Two years later, they added Rich Hanson as a partner to the RealRyder team, whose sales-marketing expertise helped launch StairMaster® Sports/Medical Products, Inc. as a pioneer in the fitness equipment manufacturing field.

Utilizing over 120 years of combined experience this team developed a superior indoor cycle designed to meet the interests and needs of elite-cyclists for both training and performance. However, the RealRyder Cycle has also revolutionized traditional indoor cycling by providing a bike that captures the functional movement and FUN of a real road ride. Our ride represents the first major design change, as it relates to the ride, since the beginning of indoor cycling in the 80s.

RealRyder International (www.realryder.com) debuted its RealRyder indoor cycle at the International Health, Racquet, and Sportsclub Association (IHRSA) trade show in March 2008. Since then the feel, fun and features of this novel bike have been recognized by health and fitness professionals, athletes, clubs, studios and rehabilitation facilities throughout the world.

# RealRyder Indoor Cycling and Education Team
## *This is how we ryde!*

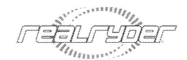

### Colin Irving

Colin Irving, cofounder of RealRyder International, a Vermont native and competitive cyclist, developed the concept of the RealRyder bike over 15 years ago. Realizing that training on the available crop of indoor-cycling tools left much to be desired, Colin envisioned an "unstationary" indoor bike that would better replicate and support the real-bike experience. Colin continues to race mountain and road bikes competitively for Team RealRyder.

### Sean Harrington

Sean Harrington, cofounder of RealRyder International, has been involved in the health/fitness industry for more than three decades. Sean opened the first Nautilus Fitness Center on the West Coast and grew the initial 4,000 square-foot location into a 38-club chain. He was the mastermind behind Heart Mate® computerized exercise equipment and later sold Heart Mate to StairMaster Sports/Medical Products, Inc. Sean continues to put full time effort into fitness product development and manufacturing.

### Rich Hanson

Rich Hanson, M.S., cofounder of RealRyder International, began his career in the health/fitness industry in 1974 by designing and building strength equipment. In 1984 he formed his own distribution company after recognizing the potential of a small company in Tulsa, OK, that manufactured a product called the "StairMaster 5000." He became a Founding Board Member of StairMaster Sports/Medical Products, Inc. Moving from an unrecognized brand to an icon in the health and fitness industry, Rich sold the company in 1996. Given his expertise, he is frequently asked to evaluate fitness products and apply research findings so the product can be improved or better understood from a scientific/evidence based perspective. Rich also coordinates the RealRyder International Sports Medicine and Health Advisory Board.

## Douglas Brooks—Director of Programming and Education

Douglas Brooks, M.S., RealRyder International's director of programming and education, is a seasoned fitness veteran with almost 30 years of experience in the industry. An ex-Ironman® triathlete, he consults as an exercise physiologist for product research and development, as well as programming for numerous fitness companies. Currently he is the Director of Athlete Conditioning at Sugar Bowl Ski Academy. The author of eight top-selling books, Douglas was inducted into the National Fitness Hall of Fame in 2008. In that same year, he was named Can-Fit-Pro's International Presenter of the Year. Brooksie and his athletes keep it real on the RealRyder cycle and in the mountains surrounding Mammoth Lakes and Truckee, California.

## Adam Reid—Lead Instructor

Adam Reid is recognized as one of the leading indoor cycling instructors in Los Angeles. His teaching passion is driven by 16 years of cycling through heavy traffic and inclement weather in Manchester, London, San Francisco and New York. Since moving to Los Angeles in 1999, he has continued to share his enthusiasm for fitness and cycling by teaching more than 5000 classes. Adam is certified by AFAA in group fitness, NASM in personal training and has multiple indoor cycling certifications. Adam teaches the fundamentals of real cycling in a format that accommodates entry level riders through champions.

## Jackie Mendes

Jackie Mendes, Brand Manager of RealRyder International LLC, is a seasoned marketing communications and brand management professional, specializing in the fitness and wellness industry. From top-selling fitness DVDs to leading infomercial programs, Jackie has written, produced and managed high profile fitness brands, bringing her creativity and deep passion for health to every project she takes on. A Certified Group Fitness Instructor with the American Council on Exercise (ACE) and Certified Cycling and Power Yoga Instructor, Jackie is proud to be a part of both RealRyder corporate and the Master Instructor Team.

# Preface

Welcome!

Once you experience the ryde and teaching methodology of RealRyder Indoor Cycling, you will never think about indoor cycle training in the same way.

Though almost every indoor cycling program has something unique to offer, the RealRyder cycle is not restricted to or limited by the bike designs of past years. Its articulating frame ("unstationary") moves under the rider and simulates a ride like you have never experienced, when compared to fixed, traditional (stationary) indoor cycles.

Since its inception in the mid-1980s, indoor cycling classes have earned a permanent slot in the weekly group exercise schedules of most health and fitness clubs, as well as in specialty cycling studios and athletic training centers. Until recently, however, the only real improvement in stationary cycle design over that period was the development of slightly sturdier bike components. That situation changed dramatically at the 2008 IHRSA Convention when the RealRyder cycle was unveiled--altering indoor bike technology forever. The innovative articulating frame allows riders to experience the natural movements of leaning, steering and balancing, which captures many of the characteristics of an outdoor ride.

The uniqueness of the RealRyder bike originates from its innovative series of linkages and pivots known as the articulating bicycle frame (ABF). The design allows the rider to move fluidly in the three natural planes of movement. With the body free to move in the sagittal, frontal, and transverse planes, riders are able to sustain an appropriate pedal cadence, while controlling the bike's sagittal, frontal, and longitudinal axes of rotation. The resulting three-dimensional movement enhances the fitness-related benefits of riding. For example, more muscle groups are activated during a ride on the RealRyder Indoor Cycle, when compared to a typical stationary bike. The large muscles of the lower body work in conjunction with the upper body and core musculature to provide a whole-body, high-calorie-burning workout. In addition, this integrated movement can also help improve riding form and postural balance.

RealRyder cycle programming, riding technique, and bike design focus on providing a "real-riding" experience. As a result of this out-of-the-box thinking an indoor cycling design evolution has occurred, one that features unlimited programming options and offers a unique riding experience that will be enjoyed by riders of all interests and backgrounds.

The RealRyder Cycling Program builds on 25-years of indoor cycling, and defines correct teaching methodology and technique. Our instructor training introduces an expanded model that allows you to teach, ride and think about indoor cycling in a different way. Cycling instructors who are used to teaching classes on traditional stationary bikes now have an opportunity to experience and teach natural bike movement.

RealRyder cycling is different. Our cycling program is different. Our bike is different. No other indoor bike has our ryde! RealRyder Cycling introduces freshness through innovation that captures substance and real-life crossover that can energize any existing cycling program.

Ryde it real. Teach it real. It's time to take the training wheels off!

# Stage 1

## Heading Out on Our Ryde

# Introduction to the RealRyder Indoor Cycling Program

The unique design and the creative programming elements set RealRyder Indoor Cycling apart from years of replication and regurgitation. *How* we teach, *why* we teach, *what* we teach, and the natural movement make us different.

The RealRyder team teaches authentic cycling as it relates to bike setup, realistic bike movement, appropriate cadence and proper form. Our coaching system is designed to "teach it real." Our program uses realistic "RydeProfiles" and drills that accommodate all ability levels. RealRyder users can maximize personal fitness and performance goals, while experiencing the joy of riding a bike. Ask a kid why he rides a bike and he will tell you, "To have fun!"

## Teaching It Real

Four key principles set the RealRyder cycling program apart:

❏ *RealRyder Cycle*

The RealRyder's articulating bike frame (ABF) moves under the rider and simulates the feel of a road bike.

❏ *Leading a RealRyde*

Our teaching system makes planning intelligent and creative indoor-cycling workouts easy. Our complete teaching approach unlocks unlimited ride possibilities.

❏ *Creating a RealRyde*

Our program is founded on an inverted triangle model (Figure 1-1). This model includes five key points (tip-to-base) that instructors can use to plan a ryde. This model depicts coaching at the macro, "big picture" level and acknowledges the importance of our moving bike frame.

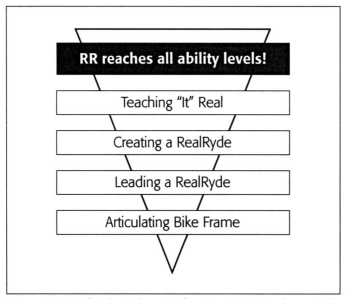

Figure 1-1. RealRyder Indoor Cycling inverted triangle model

❏ *RealRyding "Teach It Real" Philosophy*

The RealRyder team teaches it real. In fact, almost every member of our corporate and master instructor teams ride outdoors and indoors. In that regard, RealRyder cycling combines a no apologies coaching approach that teaches correct outdoor cycling principles and integrates cutting edge, science-based research into the indoor setting. The result is an effective, safe and results oriented total body riding experience that everyone can enjoy.

- *RealRyder ABF (articulating bike frame)…* The triangle's pointed "base" emphasizes the importance of core strength, balance and movement as it relates to improvement in cycling ability and overall athletic performance. The underlying teaching methodology is based on our ryde, one that no other indoor bike can replicate. Side-to-side movement, steering and stabilization challenge balance, enhance core strength and increase caloric expenditure. The pointed base of the triangle and the bike's articulating bike frame represent the foundation of the RealRyder cycling experience. This is what our ryde is built on.

- *Leading a RealRyde…* The RealRyder experience is achieved by the moving frame, bike setup, hand position, body position/form, cadence, resistance/load, intensity, and realistic riding.

- *Creating a RealRyde…* A ryde includes the science, coaching/language dimension, realistic in and out of the saddle duration, music, communication, and cueing. This represents coaching at the *micro level.* Creating a successful experience is the underlying goal for each and every ride.

  *Note:* The basic components of a RealRyder class should be based on the underlying goal(s) of the ride and participants. The results and goal attainment of the class (ryde outcome) can be manipulated by using the *cycling coach elements of variation* that are detailed in Chapter 14.

- *Teaching it real…* Our love of riding is the source of our passion. Our program teaches realistic cadence, proper technique and form. The result is an authentic, motivating bike ride and coaching style.

# 2

# RealRyder Indoor Cycling Philosophy

RealRyder Indoor Cycling philosophy is built upon:

❏ **_Indoor ryding that transfers to real cycling._** Training on the RealRyder cycle will improve outdoor riding skills and performance.

❏ **_Indoor ryding that transfers to personal fitness._** Riding indoors on the RealRyder cycle can benefit everyone by improving fitness, athletic performance and riding skills.

❏ **_Engaging riders from A to Z._** We believe that anyone from beginning rider to elite cyclist can benefit from the RealRyder experience.

❏ **_Teaching it real._** Our teaching style includes instruction in riding technique and class profile design. Our approach emphasizes what "real" cycling is all about.

❏ **_Personalized programming._** Our RydeProfiles (class structure and goals) are based on terrain, fitness level and individual goals. Using a RydeProfile class planning approach makes it easy to plan a class or teach a group of riders with mixed fitness and skill levels.

❏ **_Coach mindset._** The RealRyder cycling team believes that _how_ we teach is dependent on _who_ we are teaching. In every instance, the participants' goals and abilities are considered and take priority.

## Teach It Real

The only way to keep cycling real is to "teach it real." No excuses—no apologies and semantics aside—real cycling is real cycling. Fun, results and compliance come along for the ryde when this teaching style is implemented.

RealRyder instructor training courses and workshops build upon twenty five years of indoor cycling education. RealRyder teaching crosses over because it is pure, accurate and relevant. Instructor courses are evidence-based and supported by science.

## RydeReal: How and Why We Ryde

The truth is that teaching authentic cycling on a static bike has always been a challenge. Enter the articulating bike frame (ABF). Our ryde removes the restriction of a one dimensional bike.

When our bike, education, philosophy and unique ryde are combined the result is an experience that is engaging, authentic and fun. Ask kids why they jump on a bike and the answer won't be "To pedal!" Kids ride to have fun. The RealRyder cycle is not a pedaling machine; it is a ryding machine; it is a ryding experience. Because of this, every instructor who teaches on the RealRyder cycle can become a successful and engaging instructor, or build upon current teaching success, while still adhering to proper cycling fundamentals.

## Features and Advantages

❑ *Bike movement*…We emphasize stabilization, controlled movement and correct body position. When new riders grasp these concepts and "feel" the ryde orientation process they invariably experience an "aha" moment. At this point a new and exciting range of programming options are available to instructors and first time riders will never go back to a stationary ride.

❑ *RealRyder computer*…Incorporating output measurements into your workout can be both effective and fun. Cadence, heart rate (HR), mph, distance and caloric expenditure provide valuable feedback. Though we find this feedback useful, we believe the single most important feature an indoor cycle has to offer is related to the characteristics of the ride. Any manufacturer can put a computer on their bike, but no one has our ryde.

# 3

# Art of Ryding

The phrases "ryding-real" and "real-ryde" were coined by RealRyder bike designer and semi-pro cyclist Colin Irving. An expert cyclist, Colin realized that a more engaging and beneficial way must exist to train indoors. Bored with stationary bikes that do not allow natural cycling mechanics and frustrated with the limitation of rollers Colin gravitated toward the idea of an "unstationary bike" that would better replicate a real bike experience.

## Colin's RealRyder® Cycling Vision—the original concept

As children, we turned the pedals because we had to. It was the only way to make the bike move; we didn't love pedaling, but it was worth it. What we were rewarded with was freedom; we could lean, and steer, and coast, and *skid!* We were balancing, and thinking, and exercising—all at the same time. We loved our bikes. It was, for most of us, the first appreciation we would have for a piece of equipment that expanded our boundaries and heightened our sense of independence.

Riding a bicycle is actually a complicated procedure. Fortunately, most of us learn to ride when we are young. The diversity of controllable movement puts the bicycle into elite company when you examine and compare the physics to other methods of recreation and transportation. In fact, riding a bicycle is as close to flying as many of us will come. The real beauty of the bicycle though is that what is complicated, *feels* simple; it *feels* like unencumbered, intuitive movement. We still have to turn the pedals—it's still the only way to make the bike move, and it's still worth it.

But sometimes it rains—really hard, for days. Or we don't have time to go for an actual ride. Or we don't feel like risking our lives on the streets. So we ride one of the various indoor/stationary bikes available—a poor substitute. Now don't get us wrong. We still ride them. But they are a poor substitute!

Right? Come on—we're just sitting there turning pedals with our legs; is *this* really what we should be trying to simulate? How about the experience? How about the *feeling?* How about a few basic laws of physics governed by gravity and momentum? How about more movement, more control, and *much* more freedom!

To help you visualize our concept, imagine a bicycle connected to a frame via a series of links and pivots. The bike will rotate on two axes, like a gyroscope, allowing free movement on top of a fixed frame that sits securely on the floor.

The RealRyder cycle will provide all the health benefits of traditional stationary bikes, but, in addition, your balance, and perception, and ability to react will be constantly tested and rewarded accordingly. The result is a workout for the entire body; your arms, upper body, and core will be constantly active—adjusting, compensating and correcting. Think of a conventional bicycle: on the RealRyder cycle you are never just sitting there—your *mind* will be involved. This translates as less boredom—which means less boredom-induced-fatigue—to which we say, "Good riddance!"

The first time you ride will be a learning experience. Like a conventional bicycle, it takes body awareness and focus to understand what is happening. You will be learning a dynamic new activity, based on and very similar to the conventional bicycle, but requiring a new set of skills and reference points. The good news is you will learn quickly because the principal *fear* of riding a bicycle had been removed—the fear of falling.

On your first ride you will learn that momentum makes balancing much easier. You will learn to look forward. You will develop a smooth pedal stroke. You will appreciate the subtle nuances of free-movement, unique to the *un*stationary bicycle, and you will make the adjustments necessary to optimize speed and efficiency. Soon you will be exercising—you are past the beginner phase; you will be able to reach and sustain a high cadence while controlling the bike's natural movement. You can hold a straight line *or* lean into a long banked turn. With time and practice you will be able to navigate tight switchback turns. By adjusting your speed, steering, and balance, you will learn to find the sweet spot at any given lean angle.

The RealRyder user will be rewarded with a cycling experience unlike any other. Our bike will improve your cycling skills and technique by allowing you to experiment with more aggressive maneuvers and tactics in a fun but safe environment. Imagine pedaling at full speed (over 100 RPM) and throwing your bike into a hard right turn. You don't need to use the brakes—you're on the RealRyder bike; you can keep pedaling. The massive flywheel provides counterbalance, a smooth ride and stability. It doesn't seem possible, it doesn't look possible, but onboard it *feels* possible—and it is. You will learn how to move the RealRyder cycle through its entire range of motion confidently and securely. Like a track cyclist leaning into a steeply banked 180-degree turn, you will be able to lean—pedaling and balanced—at angles comparable to a conventional bicycle. The experience will be beyond comparison to that of riding what we now know as a stationary bike.

The involvement of both your body and your mind are what will keep you riding longer and stronger. A truly active body *and* an active mind are what set the RealRyder cycle apart from other exercise bikes. Reveling in the sensations (and awed by the sheer physics), you will glide, lean, and flow through your workout; you will be *playing* in a virtual, multi-dimensional experience. You will become one with your machine, connected to it only by your hands, feet, and seat, but feeling a much deeper connection. You will *feel* the power and the speed, you will be enthralled by the sensations, and you will be aware, and active, to your very core. You will neither forget it nor grow tired of it. I promise.

—Colin Irving

# 4

# RealRyder Indoor Cycle

We have created a unique design that allows the rider to move fluidly in the three planes of movement—sagittal, frontal and transverse. With the body free to move in these planes, riders can sustain an appropriate pedal cadence and power output, while controlling the bike's sagittal, frontal and longitudinal axes of rotation. Research shows that the resulting three-dimensional movement requires increased muscle activation of the core and increased caloric expenditure when compared to a typical stationary bike (Loy et al., 2009). The large muscles of the lower body work in conjunction with the upper body and core musculature to provide a whole-body, high-calorie-burning workout.

The integrated movements on the RealRyder cycle challenge and improve a rider's postural balance and riding form. No other bike on the market provides immediate feedback with regard to whether or not the cyclist is pedaling correctly. If the rider is not applying power smoothly throughout the entire pedal stroke, the individual will immediately notice more bike movement side-to-side. As soon as pedal technique (smooth circles) and form (upright posture, with the body's weight more over the pedals) are established, excessive lateral movement will be minimized. This immediate and nonverbal physical feedback is not only unique to the RealRyder cycle, it is essential to riders who want to take their cycling to the next level.

## Differences and Similarities Between Road Bikes and Indoor Stationary Cycles

While a number of features of indoor cycles and outdoor bikes are similar, major differences exist. The RealRyder cycle provides users with the feel of an outdoor ride. The best way for fitness enthusiasts and cyclists to fully understand this factor is to get in the saddle and experience the RealRyder difference.

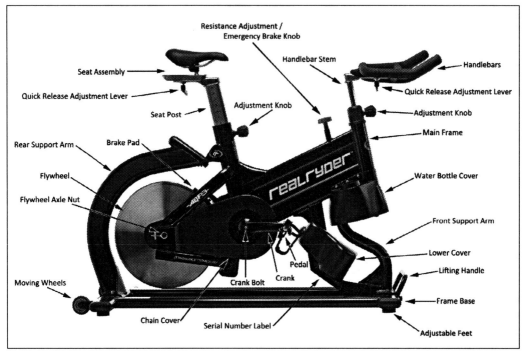

Figure 4-1. RealRyder Cycle

❑ *Resistance*...Resistance on many indoor bikes is provided by a brake caliper that pressures the flywheel. RealRyder uses a single caliper that presses down, which avoids the mechanical issues related to a dual-sided caliper that puts pressure on both sides of the flywheel. Magnetic resistance is once again growing in popularity in an attempt to gather more performance information, but we believe the feel of a realistic pedal stroke is compromised with this type of loading. Magnetic resistance offers the advantage of power measurement, but does not provide the same "on top of the gear" feel and replication of momentum that a heavy flywheel and friction resistance captures. We believe, and many indoor riders agree with us, that ride quality should never be compromised for performance feedback numbers. The key to a great riding experience rests on education, coaching style and preserving RealRyde characteristics. Nobody has our ryde.

❑ *Bike flex*...Stationary indoor bikes do not flex or bend. Even road bikes placed on stationary trainers do not feel like the real-deal. Such forced rigidity can be very hard on the bike's frame, not to mention stressful to the rider's body. In fact, riding this type of setup does not "feel right" because the forces of riding are not absorbed or dissipated by the natural movement of the bike. A combination of side-to-side bike motion and frame flex accomplishes this absorption out on the road. Outdoors, an individual strives to ride without excessive upper body movement because this represents wasted energy. As a general rule, indoor cycling on stationary fixed bikes actually requires the rider to create upper-body motion to compensate for the lack of natural side-to-side movement.

❏ *Fixed-gear and weighted flywheel*…A fixed-gear, weighted flywheel setup represents the most common system used on indoor bikes, and yet, it can also contribute to an ineffective training environment if an individual does not understand how inertia and a fixed-gear system work. Most weighted flywheels weigh between 35- and 50-pounds. A heavier flywheel creates a smoother and more realistic ride quality. Ours weighs 66-pounds.

❏ *Bike component review*…The RealRyder bike offers a quality ride that is built to last with minimal maintenance requirements. Its articulating bike frame creates a natural ride that is less stressful to the body and the bike's bottom bracket. Best of class components include pedals, crank arms, 66-pound flywheel, chain and bottom bracket.

Everyone who uses the RealRyder will appreciate that it is built to last; it is built to ryde.

# 5

# Bike Fit

Establishing a quick and accurate bike fit is essential to managing your indoor cycling class. When done poorly improper bike fit can negatively affect a participant's ride experience. Instructors should be familiar with both a basic bike fit and a more detailed micro-fit. The *basic- or quick-fit* "gets it close" and in some cases is spot on and in most cases is all you need. A *micro-fit* provides an opportunity to fine tune adjustments for those who need them. A proper bike fit is not only a matter of comfort, but also minimizes the potential for injury.

A participant who is properly fitted will be more efficient, powerful, comfortable and more likely to remain injury free on the bike. In fact, cyclists who are improperly positioned have a greater chance of experiencing overuse injuries and premature fatigue while riding. A primary goal of positioning for each rider is to adjust the bike so that the cyclist has to adapt as little as possible to the machine. In other words, it is important that the machine fits to the rider's body.

The rider's weight should be, more or less, centered over the bottom bracket. Proper positioning allows the rider to generate power efficiently by loading the legs and using appropriate resistance and cadence.

## Adjusting the Bike

The RealRyder bike uses pop-pin adjustments for seat and handlebar height, and incorporates "quick release" fore/aft adjustments for handlebar and seat position.

❑ *Seat/saddle height*

Road bikes use sliding posts, which allow for micro-adjustments. To fit a wide variety of users with ease, pop pins have become the standard.

❏ *Fore and aft seat position*

The fore/aft seat slide utilizes a quick release lever that allows for correct positioning of the feet/knees over the pedal axles. Proper positioning allows for optimal power output and minimizes risk of knee injury.

❏ *Handlebar height and fore/aft positioning*

Pop-pin adjustments allow for adequate and functional handlebar height positioning. Handlebar height positioning on an indoor bike is a matter of comfort. Recreational riders generally position the bars above saddle height because they can ride in an upright position. Conversely, riders who want specificity and transfer to road cycling will often position their seat below handlebar height to simulate a more aerodynamic position. The fore/aft adjustment allows the rider to micro adjust "the reach" which contributes to a proper bike fit.

# Basic-Fit Overview

*Note:* The seat clamp on all bikes should be set to and kept at the mid-position on the rails of the seat. <u>All bike fitting procedures assume that the seat is set at mid-position on the rails.</u> Fore/aft seat positioning changes should be made by using the slide adjustment system to ensure consistency with regard to set up from bike-to-bike.

A repeatable customized fit should be the goal for every rider. By helping students with bike setup the ride experience is enhanced and the beginnings of a professional relationship can be developed based on trust and credibility. Not only do your riders get a proper bike fit, but you are communicating to the participants from the very beginning of class that they matter and you have something to teach them.

❏ **Basic-Fit**

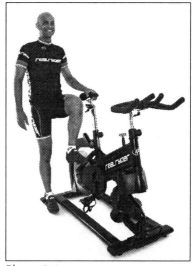

- Slide the handlebars and seat to their mid-positions. This will avoid significant adjustments later in the bike-fit process.
- *Seat/saddle height adjustment* can be determined by standing next to the bike and *off* the frame (Photo 5-1). Adjust seat height so that it is level with the top of the pelvis (e.g., head of femur or anterior iliac crest reference points). Another option would be to have the participant lift the leg that is closer to the bike saddle until the top of the thigh is parallel to the ground. The top of the thigh should be level with the top of the saddle.

Photo 5-1

- *Fore and aft seat setting is established by positioning the crank arm parallel to the ground and the pedals in the 3 o'clock/9 o'clock position* (Photo 5-2). The front knee should be aligned over or slightly behind the pedal axle.
- *Handlebar height* adjustment for indoor riding is based largely on comfort (Photo 5-3). Novice or first time riders will probably be more comfortable with the handle bar height set level with or slightly higher than saddle height. Outdoor cyclists should be encouraged to replicate the bike set up they use on their outdoor bike.

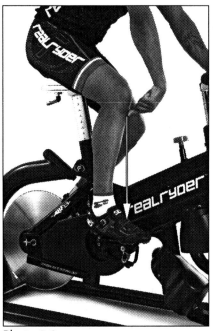

Photo 5-2

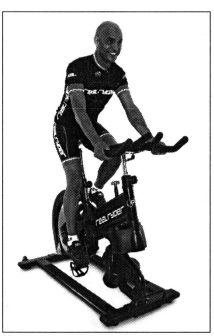

Photo 5-3

- *Handlebar fore/aft position* should be far enough forward so that the rider's knees do not hit the bar, but not so far forward that the individual is overextended or "stretched out."

This positioning should be followed up by having the participants begin pedaling in a seated position. Whether the rider is using the cages with straps or clipped-into the pedals, the widest part of the foot should be centered over the pedal axle. The rider should have a slight (i.e., 25 to 35 degree) bend in the knee when the pedal is at the bottom of the pedal stroke. The handlebar height should also be checked to ensure a comfortable position that allows the rider to maintain a slight elbow bend in any of the hand positions.

The rider should be able to ride with their hands light on the bars, hips positioned over the bottom bracket when out of the saddle, keeping their shoulders down and relaxed. The hips should not rock or tilt to either side during the pedal stroke. Be sure to confirm that the set up is correct and that the rider is comfortable.

❏ **Micro-Fit**—*Customized Setup*

As cyclists become more skilled, a fine-tuned setup becomes increasingly important for optimal performance. The following micro-fit procedure is designed to enable riders to achieve an optimal indoor bike setup.

*Note:* Riders need a partner (e.g., a coach or fellow rider) and a plumb line, which can be fabricated by attaching a heavy washer to one end of a 24-inch piece of string.

- Follow all of the steps in the *Basic-Fit* procedure to establish the starting point for micro-fit adjustments.
- *Seat/saddle height…*After setting saddle height as instructed in the basic fit, and while seated squarely in the middle of the saddle, center one heel directly over the pedal axle (Photo 5-4). Position the pedals so that the crank arms are nearly vertical, with one slightly forward of bottom dead center or the 6 o'clock position. This orientation should also align the crank arms at the same angle as the seat tube. This extended position represents the furthest point the foot will be from the hip during the pedal stroke and allows for the most extended position of the knee (Burke 2003). The rider should be able to hold this position with a fully extended knee and a level pelvis.

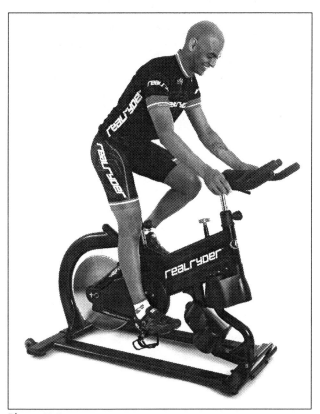

Photo 5-4

- If riders have to tilt the pelvis or move forward on the saddle to achieve this position, the seat is too high. Conversely, if the knee is flexed, the seat is too low.
- To confirm this adjustment clip into the pedals/cages and begin pedaling. The knee should be slightly flexed at about 25 to 35 degrees when the foot passes through the bottom of the stroke.

*Note:* Correct saddle height (Photo 5-5) is research-based and founded on maximum performance and injury prevention.

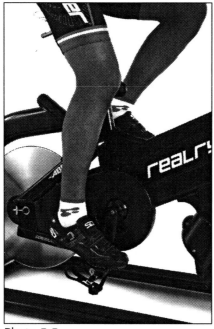
Photo 5-5

- *Fore and aft seat position…* Sit on the seat so that the sit bones (ischial tuberosities) are positioned on the widest part of the saddle (Photo 5-6a). With your feet clipped/strapped in rotate the pedals to the 3 o'clock and 9 o'clock position. Bring the crank arms *exactly* parallel to the floor. Use your partner to confirm this exact positioning. Add enough resistance so that the rider cannot move the pedals during the measurement. Maintain a centered saddle position. Place the plumb line just below the knee cap (tibial tuberosity). The vertical line should bisect the pedal axle (Photo 5-6b). If the line falls behind the pedal axle, the seat should be moved forward. If it falls in front of the axle, the seat should be moved back.
- *Handlebar fore/aft positioning…* You should be able to ride comfortably with your hands in the following positions: tops (Photo 5-7a), sides (Photo 5-7b), and aero (Photo 5-7c).

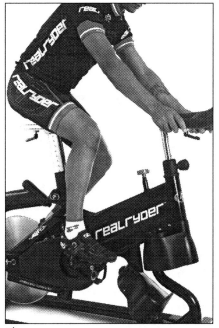
Photo 5-6a

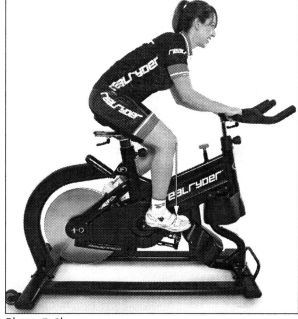
Photo 5-6b

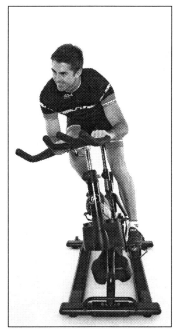
Photo 5-7a. Tops

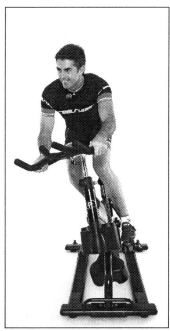
Photo 5-7b. Sides

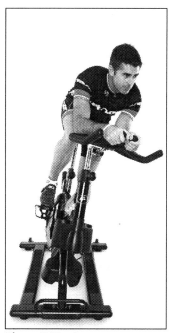
Photo 5-7c. Aero

# The Art of the Fit

**Key Point**

*"Fittings are fluid and dynamic and change over time. What works today may not work, say, two years from now. Whether it's from your body changing—you may lose or gain weight, or become more or less fit—or from getting older, your bike fit will most likely change. It's important to have it done periodically, especially if you start to feel pain or discomfort."*

—Matt Lodder, certified bike fitter

One of the more common refrains of cyclists is, "If the bike fits, you should be able to wear it!" Yes, a bike should fit like a snug-fitting riding glove. Perfect! On the other hand, the world of bike fit is not always consistent, constant, or perfect, a factor that is true for any "art." Fortunately, riders can avoid inherent imperfections in fitting a bike by working within the framework just established. As complex as bike fit can be, getting it right often comes down to the simplest "things." *Bicycling* magazine (June 2009) interviewed top bike-fit specialists and came away with a number of pearls that places the "art" and "science" into perspective, including the following insights:

- Riders who have a knee that has been bothering them for an extensive period of time should move the cleat back. This recommendation came to light after an extensive analysis of riding technique and bike-fit check and re-check. Riders who adopted this rule-of-thumb could ride faster and longer with no pain.

- According to Matt Loder, the bike fit should be started from the ground up. Initially, the shoes and cleat position should be addressed. Then, similar to the RealRyder bike fit, saddle height, saddle fore and aft, and finally, the handlebar should be dealt with. Somewhat surprisingly, even with all of this certified expertise at hand, Loder once discovered that a rider's "problem" was shoes that fit too tightly.

- Certified fitter Mike McKovich says, "You have to play to win." He breaks bike fit down into two areas: the play and the execution. The *play* entails all of the scientific stuff: seat height, seat fore and aft, stem length, and handlebar height. The *execution*, on the other hand, encompasses skills (proper pedaling, correct positioning) and physical ability (overall strength, flexibility, endurance). According to Mike, most people resort to a bike fit only when they think the *play* (technical setup) is the problem, when oftentimes, it's the *execution*. The greatest play has little impact if the situation does not involve the right athlete to execute that play. The point is reinforced by the story of a young cyclist who entered a bike race and won using a fixed-gear bike. He put to shame a number of cyclists who were riding $7,000 models. Just goes to show—no matter how good the fit or bike, riders have to have the internal fortitude and commitment to training and improving their riding skills. Put another way, "It's not the wand, it's the wizard!"

- Same bodily dimensions, different setting, according to Loder. He states, "Even if your friend is the same height, weight, and overall build as you—don't assume his bike settings are the settings you should use. His bike may ride like a dream to him, while it may ride horribly for you."
- McKovich says, "I also tell them to use their core and abdominal muscles for support. This takes weight and pressure off the hands, shoulders, and neck, and makes the bike more maneuverable."
- Ward Griffiths proclaims, "Even minor changes in handlebar reach and drop can make a huge difference in weight distribution and saddle comfort. The best advice I ever got was, if you can comfortably 'shake hands' with your brake hoods, your bike fits properly."
- According to Loder, "The best bike fit in the world means nothing, if you don't relax on the bike. Riding tense can create pain in the shoulders, neck, and low back that is unrelated to bike setup."

# Additional Details Concerning Proper Bike Fit

❑ *Proper seat height*…Research on knee pain during cycling has revealed that the correct seat height for individuals with no knee pain allows for 25 to 30 degrees of flexion of the extended leg, when the pedal is at bottom dead center. This range of knee flexion allows for adequate decompression of the knee in order to prevent anterior knee injuries. It also enables the knee to avoid the dead spot at the bottom of the pedal stroke. Seats that are too high can cause posterior knee pain (hyper-extension), whereas seats that are too low are associated with anterior knee pain (shear).

❑ *Proper bike setup tips*…Because all riders are unique, participants may need to slightly readjust the seat height after the initial setup. Any initial changes and readjustments should be undertaken in small increments. Tables 5-1 and 5-2 list helpful troubleshooting tips for proper bike setup.

❑ *Handlebar height and fore/aft position*…Upper body position is closely related to handlebar height. The upper body posture adopted by a cyclist tends to be a function of performance, comfort, experience, hamstrings and back flexibility, back problems, and the ability to rotate the hips. Beginning cyclists should start with the handlebars above seat height. As participants gain more experience and become more comfortable on the bike, they may be encouraged to lower their handlebars to the level of the tip of the seat. Riders with back problems should begin with their handlebars as high as possible.

Another important checkpoint to consider when adjusting fore and aft handlebar position is the amount of arm extension. In this regard, the rider's arm extension should be checked at the "brake hood" or "hand shake" position (Photo 5-8). If the elbows are completely extended, the bars should be moved closer to the seat. If too much bend exists in the elbow (i.e., more than slight elbow flexion), the bars should be moved away from the seat.

| Personal factors | Solution |
|---|---|
| Length of the rider's feet | Long feet have the effect of lengthening the legs beyond standard proportions. As a result, riders with feet that are long for their height may need to raise seat height. |
| Excessive soft tissue in the gluteal region | Cyclists with excessive soft tissue (i.e., fat or muscle) over their sit bones (ischial tuberosities) may need to lower the seat height. Keep in mind, however, that when the rider sits for a while, soft tissue compresses. |
| Shoe thickness | Insoles or cycling orthotics that extend under the ball of the foot have the effect of adding length to the legs. Seat height may need to be raised in these situations. |
| Space between the crotch and the seat | Adding thickness between the rider and the seat—which occurs when wearing padded cycling shorts or using a padded seat cover—effectively shortens the legs, which can require a lower seat height. |

Table 5-1. Considerations for optimal seat height position

| Problem | Correction |
|---|---|
| Hips are rocking in the seated position | The seat position may be too high. If so, the seat should be lowered in small increments until the hips remain level during pedaling. |
| Inadequate knee extension | The seat position is too low. If so, the seat should be raised in small increments until the knee-flexion range is between 10 and 40 degrees of the extended leg at bottom dead center, though 25 to 35 degrees may be optimal. |

Table 5-2. Seat height position troubleshooting tips

Complaints of numbness in the hands or pain in the neck, arms, or shoulders may indicate that the handlebars are too low. Raising them will help take pressure off of these areas and may provide a more comfortable ride. In addition, reminding participants to maintain a neutral wrist position throughout the training session will help prevent wrist discomfort and potential overuse injury. Frequent hand-position changes can limit hand discomfort and numbness.

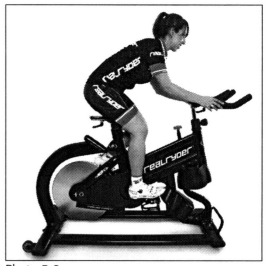

Photo 5-8

# 6

# Ryde Orientation Recipe

It is important that anyone new to the RealRyder cycle is oriented to the unique aspects and opportunities that an articulating bike frame provides. It is also useful for experienced riders to re-visit ASAP-P on a regular basis. It is fun, helps to dial in RydeTechnique and by design allows an instructor to teach a pack of riders with various ride experience while simultaneously challenging all.

Our ryde orientation starts by having the rider straddle the bike and quickly run through the ASAP-P RydeReady Drill. In less than 10-minutes any rider is completely familiar with the bike and set for a successful first experience.

The Ryde Orientation Recipe is best experienced by attending a RealRyder Indoor Cycling workshop, certification training or by clicking on an updated ASAP-P link on our website.

Following is our ASAP-P "live" workshop format outline:

## RydeReady Drill (ASAP-P)

A. **A**stride—straddling bike; lean left/right; add PLL

B. **S**teady—controlled straight line riding in the saddle

C. **A**dd a gear/proper load; transition to standing

D. **P**osture—riding positions; cadence/gear variations

E. **P**ush, Look, Lean (PLL)—lean, steer, turn head; seated/standing

    • Counter steer/lean; "setup and dive"

*Discussion Questions*

- Stabilization vs. excessive bike movement
- No bike movement vs. natural bike movement

*Repeat Drill w/ Cues; "Levels Of Success"; "Saddle Time"*

*Everything you can do on the RealRyder Cycle in 30-Seconds*

- Demonstration/Participation Repeats 5x

*Discussion Questions*

- What did you discover?
- Stabilization vs. excessive bike movement vs. movement vs. freedom
- No bike movement vs. natural bike movement

*What can you do on your indoor bike?*

*Be sure to join us for a RealRyde soon!*

# Stage 2

## RealRyder Indoor Cycling Program

# 7

# RydeTechnique—
# Hand Positions, Riding Positions
# and Riding Movements

This chapter includes several common references of a genre that essentially refers to "riding technique" or "riding form." Hand and riding positions, as well as riding movement choices define superb RydeTechnique. A proper way to ride, and *not* to ride does exist. Riding technique is either correct or incorrect—useful or not.

*Souplesse*—the French word for suppleness—is the holy grail of accomplished cyclists. The RealRyder bike is a tool that enables participants to achieve it. Hand positions, riding position, riding technique and riding movements all refer to *"form"* in the real-cycling world. Each factor contributes to "souplesse" or the style exhibited by a rider. Fluidity is what riders strive for on a bike. The RealRyder bike design allows movement to occur under the rider like a road bike, helps participants achieve that end goal, an objective that is not possible, in its truest form, on a fixed stationary bike.

The RealRyder bike enables all riders to find rhythm, coordination, balance and flow. Coordination is essential to develop motor skills. Traditional fixed-frame stationary bikes have neglected coordination because there is a limited relationship between the rider and equipment. The RealRyder is a tool that encourages and enhances coordination, balance and good riding form.

## Key Point

*Correct riding form and real-bike movement are the key elements to both indoor and outdoor cycling in terms of safety, compliance, reduced injury rate and improved riding performance.*

*Outdoor cyclists choose load, cadence and riding positions based on terrain features and fitness level. We do the same.*

RydingReal keeps it simple, familiar, effective and safe. Outdoor riding strategies tend to vary, based on an as-needed basis. For example, rough roads or cracks in the road require participants to get out of the saddle to absorb the bumps. Fatigue or stiffness from a sustained position can result in the rider moving into and out of the saddle for relief. Possible racing strategies might include standing, picking up another gear, and pedaling quicker to move up in the peloton or to power over the top of a hill.

Our indoor ride has an infinite number of riding options that can be manipulated and include terrain variations, seated/aero/standing positions, cadence and gear (resistance). Our education program complements the ride our bike offers and provides access to a new indoor riding experience.

# Hand Positions

Hand-placement ties directly to bike fit and influences riding form and biomechanics, as well as comfort. We teach three basic hand positions: sides, tops, and aero.

❑ Sides: Place the hands on the side of the bars, palms facing in, at or slightly beyond the bend in the bar (Photo 7-1).
❑ Tops: Place the hands on top of the bars shoulder width apart, palms down with a light grip (Photo 7-2).
❑ Aero (aerodynamic position): Place the hands on the forward center extensions with the forearms resting lightly on top of the bars (Photo 7-3).

The "sides" position is the key hand position providing maximum control and leverage during turning and climbing out of the saddle. The "tops" position is popular for seated climbs, recovery and can be used as a less aggressive aero-position. The "aero" position is optional and <u>only used when seated</u>. Do not overreach by placing the hands too far forward; elbows should be under the shoulders with forearms resting lightly on top of the bars (Photo 7-4). Many find it very comfortable and it is a great position to connect the rider to the bike's natural movement.

*Note:* Though traditionally unpopular on fixed stationary bikes, the aero position is not inherently uncomfortable or dangerous when your bike moves laterally—which ours does. On a fixed-frame stationary bike lateral stresses are transferred into the shoulders, hip and back.

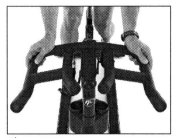
Photo 7-1

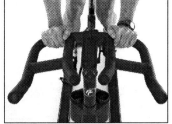
Photo 7-2

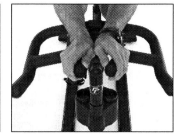
Photo 7-3

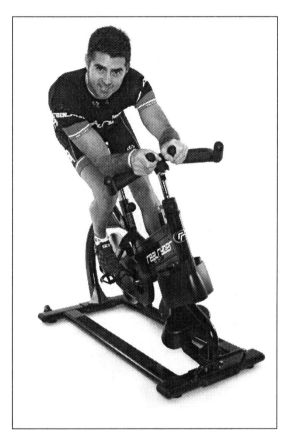
Photo 7-4

RealRyder instructors will suggest hand positions based on intensity, terrain features or ride position. But, at no point should these guidelines be considered mandatory. Riders always have permission to choose a hand position that is comfortable and appropriate.

# Ryde Fundamentals

Riders should be most comfortable in the position in which they will spend the greatest amount of time. The average endurance cyclist can spend as much as 85- to 90-percent of their ride in the saddle. When in the saddle, ride with a relaxed upper body—light on the bars, weight driving into the pedals and buttocks centered on the seat over the bottom bracket. A balanced upper body leads to a powerful, efficient pedal stroke. Arms should be slightly bent and relaxed, shoulders down, hands light on the bars. Look forward with the head, neck and spine in neutral alignment. Correct body position on the bike provides maximum comfort, performance and reduces the potential for overuse injuries.

Changing your hand placement and position on the saddle during the workout will reduce discomfort in the hands and buttocks caused by nerve compression and/or lack of blood flow.

Extreme forward positions are inappropriate, because too much weight is placed on the bars, which gives participants less control of the bike and less power output or performance capability. Riders should "load the pedals" by keeping their hands "light on the bars."

# Unlocking the Ryde

*Take what the bike gives you. Take what the bike gives you. Take what the bike gives you.*

The non-verbal, constant and immediate feedback provided by the RealRyder can be a powerful teacher. Our ride rewards good form and proper pedal stroke. Poor positioning and faulty technique can restrict movement or cause too much side-to-side motion.

Encourage the participant to be patient and maintain a dialogue with the bike. The conversation is focused on movement and feedback. A dynamic athletic experience is never fully realized during the first outing. Any activity that depends on interaction with your equipment—cycling, skiing, surfing—requires patience and openness to the feedback the equipment is providing. Similarly, developing this relationship and maintaining a dialogue with your RealRyder bike never gets old.

# Ryding Position

Initial considerations with regard to body position (seated, standing, aero) include spinal position, foot position, proper positioning in the saddle, and knee position during the pedal stroke.

❑ *Spinal position*…Maintaining a neutral spine reduces accumulative tension and fatigue in the lower back. Riders who have a difficult time maintaining a traditional riding position may have tightness in their lower back, hip flexors, and/or hamstrings, in addition to weak abdominal musculature. Instead of riding with a protracted shoulder girdle and rounded (flexed) spine, recreational riders should be encouraged to keep their spine neutral, raise the handle bars above seat height and work on increasing low-back and hamstrings flexibility. Competitive cyclists usually assume flexed and protracted positions, because they understand that while this posture can be stressful, it is part of the specificity of riding and results in a more aerodynamic position. Participants who are looking for health and fitness benefits, rather than a competitive racing edge, should be encouraged to assume a more comfortable ride position.

❑ *Foot position*…Proper foot position is achieved when the widest part of the foot is directly over the pedal axle (refer to Chapter 5, Bike Fit). In addition, the foot should be kept relatively flat through the pedal stroke. Chapter 9 provides more details on pedal-stroke dynamics.

❑ *Proper positioning in the saddle*…Cyclists spend most of their time in the saddle so proper setup is important for comfort. As a rule, the sit-bones (ischial tuberosities) should be positioned on the widest part of the saddle, hands lightly gripping the bars, elbows are slightly flexed, shoulders are down and relaxed, and the wrists are neutral. Three key coaching tips include: keep the elbows soft, ride relaxed and stay light on the bars.

❑ *Knee position during the pedal stroke*…Driving the knees forward, not outward or inward, is essential to knee health and power output. While pedaling drive the knees forward keeping the hip, knee and ankle aligned; visualize a narrow corridor for each leg where the knee does not touch either wall. Another useful cue is to have the rider aim the knee toward the second toe. This prevents the knee from straying too far in or out.

Three ryding positions—seated, standing, and aero—create the foundation for all RydeProfiles and workout variations.

## ❑ *Seated Flat or Seated Climbing*

• *Seated flat—minimal-to-heavy resistance; moderate-to-high cadence*

RydingReal equates to a significant amount of time in the saddle. There should not be a rush to get out of the saddle—*seated riding is the cornerstone of cycling* (Photo 7-5). The key is to find a balance between riding in both a seated and a standing position. Keep it real and the riding experience will quickly produce buy-in and committed riders who are becoming proficient cyclists, but still having fun.

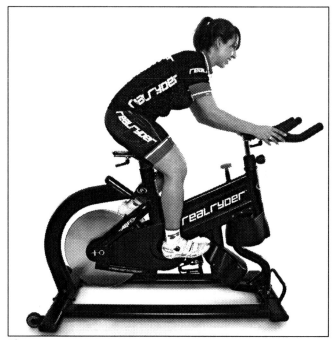

Photo 7-5

• *Seated climbing—moderate-to-heavy resistance; moderate-to-lower rpm*

Participants can engage in seated climbing technique that results in a pedal resistance increase and a slower pedal cadence. This higher-intensity technique promotes lower-body strength and endurance and increases the demand on the body's cardiorespiratory system. Shifting the buttocks to the back of the seat maximizes pedaling efficiency, especially when the hill is steep and you cannot stay "on top of the gear." This "shifting of the hips" slightly back allows for more recruitment of the gluteal muscles and provides a welcome relief from a centered or slightly forward seated position. The hands can be placed wider on the handlebars ("sides") to promote stability and to open the chest for increased breathing capacity. The grip should be light on the bars, with the fingers relaxed. If riders slip to the front of the saddle to gain leverage, they can move their hands to the top of the bars ("tops") and pull the bike toward them as they pedal. Keeping a neutral spine and a relaxed upper body are important reminders, since the level of intensity increases during a seated climb (Photo 7-6). Participants can visualize riding a moderate-to-steep incline, while using the seated climbing technique.

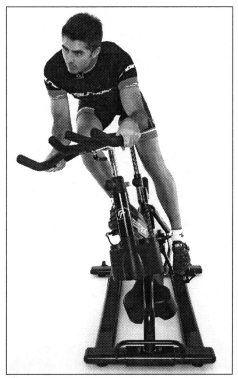
Photo 7-6

### ❑ *Standing Flat Riding or Standing Climbing Riding Positions*

• *Standing flat—light-to-moderate-to-heavy resistance; moderate to slow rpm*

Coming out of the seat into a standing position during cycling requires that a light-to-moderate resistance be maintained on the pedal to counteract the rider's body weight. Maintaining resistance on the flywheel will facilitate the rider's efforts to keep complete control of the pedals. In the standing position, the rider's body weight should be centered over the pedals, with the hands lightly gripping the handlebars in a wide or "sides" position. The hips should be kept behind the shoulders, the spine should remain neutral and the upper body should be relaxed (Photo 7-7).

The standing flat position releases tension in the lower back and shoulders and facilitates breathing. With each down stroke the hips and shoulders should be kept level and facing forward.

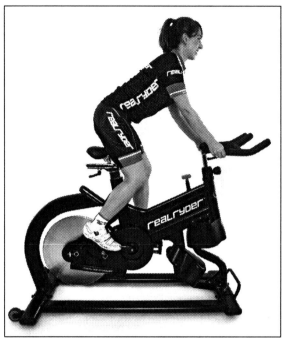

Photo 7-7

## Key Point

*Core stability development in this position is ideal because you lose your key anchor point—the buttocks in contact with the saddle. Core activation and coordination requirements become very pronounced when you stand. Though you only have one less point of contact with the bike, controlling the bike's movement through foot and hand contact only is much more challenging. This is where balance, strength and coordination all come together.*

Questions that often come up include, "Should I get out of the saddle on a flat road?" "How often and for how long?" and "What do road cyclists do?" A roadie might get out of the saddle for brief periods of time when on a flat road to use different muscles, "stretch out," or "lengthen" the legs, and to generally give the body a break from a prolonged seated position. The rider might even click up a gear or two to accelerate. Getting out of the saddle on the flats is appropriate for both recovery and race strategies. It is an acceptable technique for indoor riding because it often provides a welcome change-of-pace. Though hard-core riders tend to appreciate the pay-off of disciplined seated riding, recreational cyclists typically prefer a more varied ride with shorter intervals between seated and climbing postures.

When riders stand the bike motion should remain controlled, quiet and natural. Standing hip angle is about the same as seated hip angle, and changes depending on load, but should never be completely upright. Though "pressuring heavy" on the bars should be avoided, the shoulders should not be excessively back and over the hips, either. Teaching an upright standing posture with only the rider's fingertips on the bars is incorrect. "Finger tip riding" leads to an inefficient pedal stroke and mechanical stress to the knees. Smooth and round revolutions disappear as riders bounce off the bottom of the pedal stroke. No sound reasoning exists to teach this contrived posture. In fact, on the road this technique would make it impossible to control the bike and it would be outrageously dangerous.

## Key Point

*Keeping your center of gravity—weight into the pedals and light on the bars—is a fundamental cue that cannot be overstated.*

Minimize the amount of time devoted to long periods of standing on the flats with high cadence, since it is not specific to cycling and not particularly enjoyable for a recreational rider. Seventy-five to ninety-five rpms is realistic and manageable for most riders. Participants should be encouraged to experiment with finding their own cadence and resistance to optimize their ride experience.

*Note:* Refer to Chapter 12, *Energy Zone Training,* for guidance on recommended intensity.

Many riders shift weight forward onto the bars when standing on the flats or during a climb because they don't have the leg strength or coordination to turn the pedals. Over time, short-duration standing flat or climbing drills—"after clicking up a gear or two"—can improve leg strength in standing positions. When transitioning from seated to standing the rider should ALWAYS stay close to the saddle which will keep their weight centered over the bottom bracket.

## Key Point

*The art of standing—An experienced rider hovers slightly above the nose (front) of the saddle feeling the "wind of the saddle" brushing the inside of the legs. This breath of space and "contact" is virtually nonexistent, subtle and developed over time—but always present!*

Any hitch (e.g., a "flat spot") in pedal stroke fluidity indicates that the rider is not balanced over their pedals and is incorrectly positioned on the bike.

• *Standing climbing—moderate-to-heavy resistance; slow to moderate rpm*

During a standing climb, the rider's hands should be placed in the "sides" position or slightly forward. Arms and torso length ultimately determine where the hands are placed. Body weight should always be centered over the bottom bracket and weight is "down into the pedals." For example, if reaching too far forward on the bars forces the rider into an overly flexed-forward position or pulls the hips forward, the hands may need to be placed closer to the rider's body. The same principles that hold true for standing flat riding are appropriate for standing climbs.

A standing climb can represent a high-intensity effort or an easy recovery. Higher intensity climbing promotes lower-body strength/endurance, core strength, coordination and increases demand on the cardiorespiratory system. During an aggressive climb the bike moves naturally side-to-side with each pedal stroke and the shoulders are level. The standing climb position is also ideal for developing core strength and stability. Leaning and steering may be utilized during standing climbs. But, it is a good idea to limit this "advanced drill" to shorter durations (e.g., 5-6 revolutions) until the rider can sustain longer leans and turns with good form.

## ❑ *Seated/Standing Combination and "Jumps"*

Regardless of resistance (gear) or cadence, a number of riding options exist when individuals move from seated to standing postures. How do you change the ride on an indoor cycle? You get in and out of the saddle, change the load, vary the cadence and on the RealRyder you can lean and steer the bike. Moving in and out of the saddle is often referred to as "combos" or "jumps." Participants alternate between seated and standing positions, and simultaneously overcome added resistance to power out of the saddle. "Jumps" are used in outdoor riding to power over a hill without dropping a gear (decreasing resistance), to close or create a gap (distance between riders), to break away from the peloton or group of riders an individual wants to challenge, or simply to create a race-attack strategy.

At RealRyder we focus on authentic riding which does not support consecutive high repetition jumps. Simply, we teach RealRyding and ryde with intent and purpose that ties to our RydeProfile (terrain challenges). Teaching "real" on an articulating bike provides many more teaching variables that relate to the characteristics of road riding. Repeated jumps are *not authentic.* Responding to and controlling our bike's natural movement—balancing, leaning, steering—makes obsolete this contrived drill based on the limitations of traditional stationary bikes. RealRyder instructors often comment about how they are too busy leading the ryde to be sidetracked by trivial pursuits.

Transitioning from seated to standing should be used realistically (sparingly) to respond to the RydeProfile and interact with other riders. Quickly popping on and off the seat increases the likelihood of momentum driving the rider's actions—instead of applying muscular force effectively with the legs. The key to performing this transition is appropriate load, correct cadence and maintaining a smooth application of power which avoids any "flat spots" in the pedal stroke.

Grip the bars lightly and use them to help you balance and fine tune your position on the bike when lifting out of the seat. The hands should be shoulder-width in the "sides" position, the spine neutral, and the upper body relaxed throughout the duration of the stand-and-sit transition. Effective seated-to-standing-to-seated riding requires a high degree of leg strength, core stabilization, balance and coordination. Adding leaning and turning while standing should be undertaken for short durations initially to ensure the highest degree of success and fun.

# Fundamentals of Indoor Cycling

Everything that you have learned about indoor cycling to date that is validated by scientific information still holds true. Cadence/resistance variations, seated or standing positions, rolling hills, pyramids, "running," accelerations, intervals, closing the gap, creating a gap, break-aways or jumps—all collectively encompass a form of training that is relevant to cycling. Couple this accepted methodology with our articulating frame and become part of the RealRyde that has exponentially advanced the indoor cycling experience.

**Key Point**

*The limitations of a traditional (stationary) indoor bike have long been accepted despite the lack of specificity of transfer to real cycling or even basic functional movement.*

A variety of cadence, resistance and seated/climbing combinations work effectively as teaching strategies and represent a basic manipulation of drills and RydingTechnique that often does not tie to authentic riding strategy and class planning. Many of these drill combinations are organized into "traditional" riding drills for the instructor in Chapter 14, *Creating A Ryde—Planning Your Class Workouts.* These drills make it relatively easy for instructors to create varied indoor-cycling classes. However, our recommended way of planning a class rests on the "RydeProfile" which is detailed in Chapter 14.

**Key Point**

*Using a RydeProfile planning strategy moves away from memorizing drills for the sake of having a drill and moves toward ryding that responds to real terrain profile challenges. The RydeProfile methodology is driven by purpose and intent and it is quick and easy to use.*

- *Interval Training (IT), sprints, accelerations and speed work.* Interval Training involves some combination of seated/standing positions and the manipulation of cadence toward high or low rpms and heavy or light resistance. A series of exaggerated efforts and recoveries allows the rider to work on cardiorespiratory fitness, coordination and strength. Additional detail is provided in Chapter 12, *Energy Zone (EZ) Training.*
- *Speed work or sprinting.* Sprinting or speed work is a high-intensity technique that challenges the rider's ability to pedal quickly, while still maintaining smooth, fluid pedal strokes without bouncing in the seat or generating excessive lateral movement. The rider's hands are in a wide "sides" position on the handlebars, with the spine neutral and the upper body relaxed. It is important for riders to keep adequate resistance on the flywheel to avoid losing form, to control the pedals and keep power output high, which "moves the bike forward." Sprinting is an advanced skill that requires practice to develop.

Core control is essential to sprinting effectively on the RealRyder or an outdoor bike and can be developed by riding our bike. The RealRyder bike simulates the degrees of freedom cyclists have on a road bike. It allows the rider to move in sagittal, frontal, and transverse planes and not only requires, but develops proper core muscle activation, balance and coordination.

# Sprints or SPRINTS?

All-out SPRINTS typically occur at the end of races with one rider claiming victory—arms stretched overhead in celebration. Cycling literature refers to true sprints as an all out effort, but let us not forget this is in reference to competitive cyclists who have the skill and are prepared to risk all to win a race. Approach this tactic with caution and remind your riders that before they consider throwing their arms in the air for a victory salute they should remember that they are riding a fixed gear bike. No free-wheeling means no celebration indoors (i.e., arms overhead) until they have the flywheel/pedal stroke under control or they have shut it down with their emergency brake.

"Sprinting" is commonly referenced as any drill or strategy that bumps up intensity by using load and/or cadence increases. Sprints, all out "attacks" or "intense accelerations" can occur at any point in the ride. This effort can last 30 meters, 30-seconds or a few seconds and can involve a situation in which the rider *can* recover "on the ride" after backing off. It is important to note that a short-surge or all-out sprint can occur several times, even in a race that exceeds 100 miles. Whether it is a "sprint," or a "SPRINT," be certain your riders understand what you expect and that the rider has the capability to control the experience.

# Proper Breathing and Posture Checks Impact Ryding Form

A number of variables can impact an individual's overall RydingTechnique and/or the person's ability to sustain form and power.

*Proper breathing.* Cycling is highly dependent on oxygen delivery. All other factors being equal, riders who breathe efficiently will outperform those who do not. Chest breathing should be avoided. Even though shallow breathing brings oxygen into the lungs it is not energy efficient. Chest breathing (expanding and lifting the ribs using the intercostal muscles) requires a higher heart rate and greater oxygen cost when compared to "deep belly" or "diaphragmatic" breathing.

Diaphragmatic respiration helps to move air deep into the lungs, where a greater surface area exists for the exchange of oxygen between the blood and the alveoli. During inhalation, the lower rib cage expands, and the abdomen slightly protrudes. During exhalation, the lungs recoil, the diaphragm lifts and the abdominals contract. This scenario entails the most efficient form of respiration in terms of oxygen cost and efficient oxygen exchange.

To conserve energy, ride relaxed and optimize riding form—riders must learn how to breathe deeply, while at the same time keeping their core muscles engaged. Proper breathing occurs during the respiration cycle when riders learn to let their rib cage and abdomen expand on inhalation and contract during exhalation. Mastering this technique lies in the art of learning how to relax and breathe deeply on the inhalation while still being able to retain a cat-like readiness to attack or respond.

*Posture breaks.* A sustained forward-flexed position of the spine can become uncomfortable. Optional on-bike breaks can be offered during class to alleviate any discomfort associated with cycling posture. Some riders may *choose* to maintain a cycle specific posture that has a high cross-transfer to road riding (e.g., time trials) and not abandon their ride form at any point during the ride—foregoing posture breaks to develop ride specific conditioning.

# 8

# Questionable Indoor Cycling Form and Technique

Instructors have their own ideas with regard to what the riding experience should be based on their cycling and teaching background. What we believe to be true is that the simplicity and pureness of cycling, without unnecessary or unsafe distraction, represents the joy of riding. Because cycling has its inherent virtues, nothing needs to be fabricated or exaggerated simply for the sake of variety. Cycling is an engaging physical and mental experience—Why change that?

Instructors are constantly challenged to stay current and accurate as they sort through a myriad of conflicting information. We subscribe to the principle that "everything we know about cycling today may be wrong," which gives us the freedom to consider change that is justified. RealRyder Indoor Cycling takes a special interest in teaching the most appropriate, up-to-date and authentic cycling information.

None of us are perfect, and most of us can look back and chuckle about what we used to teach. But, rather than focus on what we did not know but now do—one must admire those who implement change that is warranted and refuse to continue teaching information that is inaccurate or inappropriate. This chapter (and Chapter 7, RydeTechnique) is about moving on and upgrading our teaching approach for indoor cycling.

The potential list of questionable riding techniques continues to expand. This chapter highlights several misrepresentations of authentic riding. These are distortions that

## Key Point

*If it is not relevant to outdoor cycling and does not make you a better athlete, why do it?*

undermine the principles of accepted cycling fundamentals. Understanding why each approach is scientifically suspect reinforces the RealRyder message—Keep The Ryde Authentic.

❑ *Too fast/too slow*...Proper cadence and resistance selection allows every rider to achieve the intensity level that is appropriate for that day's training session and contributes to proper body position and pedal stroke. The RealRyder instructor training program contains numerous references concerning the why, how, and "the good, the bad, and the ugly" of out of control pedaling (too light) or extremely heavy resistance. Riders must find the balance between slowing down their legs, "feeling the road," using the right gear/resistance and creating power output—while maintaining proper form. Chapters 7 and 10, *RydeTechnique* and *Cadence and Resistance* provide an in-depth discussion of proper cadence, resistance selection and riding form.

❑ *Frozen riding, "freezes," or isolations*...As part of this problematic approach that is done traditionally on stationary bikes the rider is instructed to ride with no upper-body movement. This technique mandates that natural movement be largely eliminated which is in direct opposition to correct bike form. While a little shoulder drop side-to-side is common on a fixed stationary bike to compensate for the lack of frame movement, it is not necessary with a natural side-to-side movement like the RealRyder bike provides. The shoulders should remain level throughout the ride on our cycle, which also holds true for outdoor riding, because the bike moves under the rider in a natural rhythm.

❑ *Upright quad running*...(Photo 8-1) This technique involves standing as upright as possible and moving the weight forward of the saddle and onto the bars. Sooner or later, the rider's quads, arms, and upper traps scream out in agony. But, this pain has nothing to do with riding properly or optimizing fitness. Furthermore, the quad running position contradicts what science teaches us about proper riding form and body position. Standing extremely upright and balancing on your fingertips is also off target and actually dangerous on the road as it is impossible to control your bike.

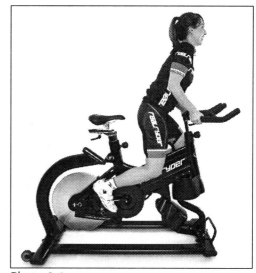

Photo 8-1

❏ *Low-rider, minis, or squat riding…*(Photo 8-2) The goal is to assume a low, upright position that is forward of the saddle; up and down movement may be incorporated but the end result is the same. This positioning places considerable shear forces (mechanical stress) across the knee because of the load (resistance). When performing squat riding, an element of speed is often introduced and further increases the risk versus benefit factor. Everything about this posture is totally contrived.

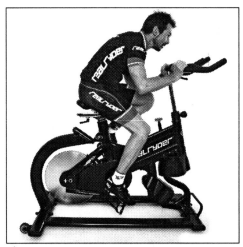

Photo 8-2

❏ *Push back or "riding the back wheel"…*(Photo 8-3) Cyclists know the exhilaration of riding a gradual hill at a challenging and ever-increasing work load. As the workload (the incline of the hill) slightly increases, rather than standing, riders can maintain cadence and handle the increase in resistance by *subtly* pushing back in their saddle a quarter or half inch. If they push back too far, beyond the back edge of their saddle, they are "riding the back wheel." This is just plain awkward, inefficient and dangerous.

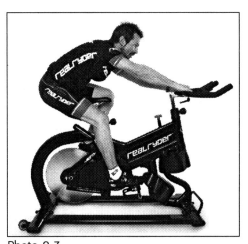

Photo 8-3

❑ *Pulling in the abs*…Core control while riding should not focus on a sustained core brace or sucking the naval toward the spine. Doing so goes against efficient "belly" or deep diaphragmatic breathing technique. Bracing the core continually or trying to keep the belly pulled in does not allow efficient breathing—from an oxygen cost standpoint—and limits the availability of oxygen by increasing the workload of the diaphragm and intercostal muscles. Belly breathing also increases oxygen saturation of the blood and helps improve the exchange of oxygen and metabolic byproducts. On the ride a cyclist should push out or distend the belly as they inhale while still activating the core enough to control and balance the bike.

❑ *On and off*…(Photo 8-4) This procedure involves a "jump" technique in which riders are instructed to "pull" themselves from the seat, load their weight on the bars, spin until their quads burn and "throw" themselves back into the seat. No core control, no loading or powering out of the saddle, no balance over the pedals and bottom bracket, no scientific basis—everything about this is all wrong. This practice defies any logical reasoning other than "variety for the sake of variety."

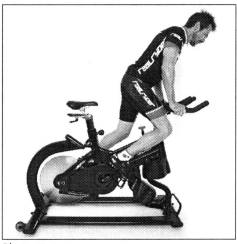

Photo 8-4

❑ *Combos or jumps*…While pedaling, riders alternate between seated and standing. Under certain conditions jumps can be fun, challenging and effective. Moving in and out of the saddle correctly can help riders increase leg strength, as well as improve their ability to transition into and out of the saddle against heavier resistance or a "bigger gear." The practice of jumping (e.g., popcorn jumps) can easily be abused which can lead to poor form, unwanted stress on the body's joints and an elevated risk of injury. If jumps are employed the number of jumps should be limited, a sound reason for "jumping" should be established, proper load should be used and riders should focus on pedal stroke and maintain proper position when driving out of the saddle.

❑ *Riding "seatless"…* This "practice" refers to a rider lowering the seat of the bike to render it unusable or even resorting to the extremes of removing the seat and post from the frame. The most important riding position in cycling is seated and therein lies the irony. It is poor coaching to force riders to stay out of the saddle for unusually long periods of time and expect them to maintain proper form, cadence and load. Cyclists develop pedaling efficiency, endurance and power which occurs in *both* the seated and standing positions. Eliminating one of these options is unacceptable. Riders create power when power is needed and move in and out of the saddle when needed—it is that simple.

❑ *Everything but RealRyding…* This genre encompasses almost anything you might find in a three-ring circus. This includes forced riding postures that are low, stretched out, or otherwise inappropriate; push-ups or "pulsing"; the use of hand weights; crunches seated or standing; and randomly changing from one hand position to another. All of these manufactured variations have no authentic connection to cycling, can be unsafe and detract from proper body positioning and pedaling mechanics.

**Key Point**

*Keep it pure. RydeReal!*

# 9

# Science of Cycling

Traditional indoor cycling programs are conducted on rigid, stationary cycles. RealRyder cycling introduces the rider to more functionally dynamic training. The pivot points and linkage of the RealRyder bike allows an actual turning movement (i.e., a rotation through a longitudinal axis) that is similar to what is experienced on a road bike. In addition, the body of the bike tilts side-to-side, which enables it to sway in the frontal plane through a sagittal axis. Furthermore, the rotation of the handlebars and the tilt of the frame are resisted by the bike's internal recoil mechanism, which challenges the musculature of the upper-body and core.

The innovative characteristics of the RealRyder cycle allow the rider to experience several positions of dynamic imbalance, which creates a training environment that is rich in balance-enhancing opportunities. Because of the design of the RealRyder cycle—pedaling force mechanics, pedaling technique and riding form closely approximates a ride on the open road. This freedom greatly impacts ride mechanics when compared to traditional indoor stationary bikes (Chapter 7, RydeTechnique). This is where science matches up perfectly with our design.

## Applied Anatomy and Biomechanics

Detailed electromyography (EMG) studies have identified the primary cycling muscles of the leg (Figure 9-1), including the sequence of the firing muscle fibers that are involved in the activity, as well as the intensity and duration of the muscular action. Several major lower-extremity muscles help move the bike forward by powering hip extension. The gluteus maximus and biceps femoris (hamstrings group) play a substantial role in hip extension, from 0-degrees at top dead center (TDC) to 180-degrees at bottom dead center (BDC). The rectus femoris, vastus medialis and vastus lateralis—the key extensors of the knee—are active from 0- to 75-degrees, and during the last 90-degrees of the recovery, which also helps to flex the hip and unload the pedal during the recovery phase. It is important to unload the pedal so that the rider does not interfere with the power phase of the pedal stroke. The primary function of the hip extensors is to extend the hip in the propulsion or power phase of the pedal stroke. While hip extension is critical to the pedal stroke, knee extension and flexion are also important in the production of force during cycling and for achieving a smooth stroke (Burke 2002).

*Muscle Group-Activity Periods During a Complete Pedal Revolution* (Figure 9-1, Faria and Cavanagh 1978) provides a detailed visual representation of pedal stroke muscle activity.

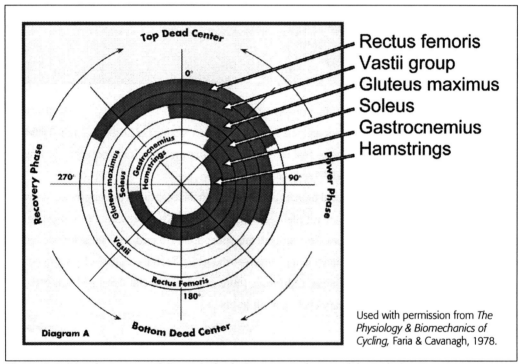

Used with permission from *The Physiology & Biomechanics of Cycling*, Faria & Cavanagh, 1978.

Figure 9-1. Muscle group activity periods during a complete pedal revolution

***Power and the pedal stroke***…A bike is powered by a rider's legs and feet, which drive the crank arms. A rider's pedal stroke is a fixed circular pattern, but a variety of pedal forces are applied throughout the pedal stroke. This changing pedal/foot position results in an "ankling pattern." An optimal ankling pattern does exist (see Figures 9-2 and 9-3) and in turn results in optimal power output.

The muscle group-activity pattern illustrated in Figure 9-1 shows that most of the force in a pedal stroke is generated from 12 to 6 o'clock (i.e., during the power phase). Although the recovery phase generates little force, it is still essential to a smooth pedal stroke, but still supports "unloading the pedal," which is contrasted with "pulling up the pedal," during the recovery phase. The gluteus, which extends the hip, "fires" for a relative short time, but is active for almost 75% of the power phase. The vastii group (quadriceps) is similarly active, whereas the hamstrings remain active longer through the end of the power phase. It is important to note that "extending" the power phase—in other words, finishing this phase—is critical.

***Recovery phase***…A number of muscles contribute to a smooth pedal stroke and the all-important power phase. But, the biggest misconception as it relates to the pedal stroke is that riders flex the knee and "actively pull up the pedal" during the recovery phase (6 to 12 o'clock). Contrary to popular belief, the hamstrings group "goes quiet"—exhibits little muscle activity—as the pedal moves past bottom dead center. It is the force created by the opposite leg beginning the power/push phase that actually flexes the knee at this point—not an actual contraction of the hamstrings.

These facts emphasizes how important it is for the recovery leg to "stay out of the way" of the pushing leg during the power phase. Riders should "stay just ahead of the power phase," so that the power phase is not inhibited by a "slow" recovery phase leg. Instead, during the recovery portion of the pedal stroke, un-weighting or unloading the pedal is the focus, which is in contrast to actively pulling up the pedal. RealRyder cycling teaches the rider to pull the *leg* up to unweight the pedal, and NOT to pull up the pedal. As one leg enters into the recovery half of the pedal cycle, the basic objective is to have the recovery leg stay ahead of pedal speed so that it has no deceleration effect on the power phase. The rider must avoid any counter-resistance being created as the opposite leg drives into its power phase.

**Key Point**

> *To better comprehend pedaling mechanics it is important to understand that while riders will be "pulling up the leg," they will not be pulling up the pedal during the pedal stroke. Instead, the rider simply unloads or unweights the pedal by pulling up the leg. This action keeps the recovery leg ahead of pedal speed.*

# Pedaling Force Mechanics During a Pedal Revolution

The pattern of force during the pedal stroke begins at top dead center and is applied throughout the pedal cycle (Figure 9-2). Force output and the angle of the foot during the pedal stroke continually change. Peak force occurs at 90-degrees or when the pedal is at 3 o'clock. Significant force is still applied to the bottom of the stroke or at 6 o'clock—a scenario that cyclists attach importance to by "trying to stretch the crank arm,"—as they aggressively drive the pedal down through and finish the power phase with an exclamation point.

Research has shown that the most effective force production occurs when force is applied perpendicular to the crank. Much of the force is downward and forward over the top (0-7 in Figure 9-2) and downward and backward for the remainder of the pedal stroke. Little, if any, "pulling up" force exists during the recovery phase. This fact reinforces the concept of un-weighting the pedal by pulling up the recovery leg (not the pedal) so that the power phase is not inhibited. Cyclists should try to make the propulsive phase of the pedal cycle as long as possible—"stretch the crank arm." This factor is the underlying premise behind visualizing the creation of a "longer" power phase. The application message in this instance is to "finish the power phase." In other words, cyclists should not stop applying force at any point during the power phase. Finish it!

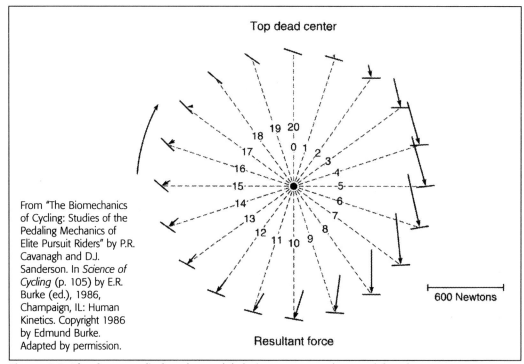

Top dead center

From "The Biomechanics of Cycling: Studies of the Pedaling Mechanics of Elite Pursuit Riders" by P.R. Cavanagh and D.J. Sanderson. In *Science of Cycling* (p. 105) by E.R. Burke (ed.), 1986, Champaign, IL: Human Kinetics. Copyright 1986 by Edmund Burke. Adapted by permission.

600 Newtons

Resultant force

Figure 9-2. The force applied to the pedal during one complete pedal cycle

It is impossible to maintain equal force output throughout the pedal stroke, even though a smooth and consistent pedal stroke can be established. Research provides a clear picture of the most efficient (correct) and least mechanically stressful technique. "Pulling up" in the pedal stroke can mean different "things" to different people. Though the hip flexors work to pull up the leg in the recovery phase, the key is to unweight the pedal so that the power stroke can drive a more "passive" recovery. But, to do so, the recovery leg, must be active to stay ahead of pedal speed. The basic goal—expressed another way—is to simply get the weight of the recovery leg off the pedal. Figure 9-2 indicates that force applied at the bottom of the stroke is not totally efficient. The most efficient direction of applied force to the pedal occurs from about 2 o'clock to 4 o'clock, which is consistent with the greatest pedal forces shown in Figure 9-2. Unloading the pedal during the recovery phase can negate any "drag effect" on the power phase of the pedal stroke.

Power output is most pronounced during the power phase from 0-degrees (12 o'clock) to 135-degrees (about 4 o'clock). Power output significantly decreases at 180-degrees (6 o'clock). The sweet spot of the stroke in terms of efficiency and power is arguably between 2 o'clock and 4 o'clock because optimal muscle recruitment and force angles occur here.

**Key Point**

*Unloading the pedal during the recovery phase minimizes inefficiency and maximizes the power phase of the pedal stroke.*

Pulling up the pedal can decrease power, waste energy and lead to poor pedaling mechanics. Because of the greater force produced in the power phase of the pedal cycle, the pedal in the recovery phase is moving more quickly than the leg can pull it. This results in a futile attempt to "pull up the pedal" and hinders optimal pedal force application. We have intentionally been redundant in explaining this concept; it is that important. With proper resistance, teaching the feel of pedaling correctly can be accomplished on an indoor bike.

## Pedal Foot Position and Proper Ankling Pattern

The ball of the foot should be positioned directly over the pedal axle. Many cyclists erroneously believe that the heel should be dropped as they pedal over top dead center and that the foot should be pointed at the bottom of the pedal stroke. An ankling pattern that exhibits a low-heel position from 30-degrees before and after the top of the pedal stroke or utilizes an extreme ankle (toe pointed downward) position anywhere in the pedal stroke represents incorrect and inefficient form. The pedaling force concepts discussed previously (Figure 9-2) are based on sound research as it applies to proper foot positioning. If a rider strays from the ankling pattern exhibited in Figure 9-3 (b), the individual is pedaling incorrectly.

When riders experience incorrect ankle-alignment patterns or a dominant heel-down or toe-down position through most of the pedal stroke, their bike fit should be checked. Also, it is difficult to pedal with a toe-down position when riding with enough resistance. As Figure 9-3 (b) indicates, the foot/pedal is in an almost flat position through most of the circle pattern, which is why a flat-foot position is recommended for pedaling. In other words, take a complicated process and simplify it. When the foot and pedal are at their flattest in the pedal stroke, this is where the most force in the power phase is exerted.

High-speed filming and pedal-force studies confirm that foot position varies from almost horizontal in position 3 to slightly heel-down in position 6, to a maximum toes-down position in position 16 in Figure 9-2. It should be noted that the toes-down position is not aggressive, and certainly is not so extreme that it would be considered as "toes-pointed." Research supports the fact that a good cue to achieve a proper foot position while cycling is to encourage a "relative flat foot" through the pedal stroke.

## Key Point

*As a general rule, cueing a relatively flat foot will create a desired foot position or ankling pattern throughout the pedal cycle without having to over-coach a rider.*

An ankling pattern that is anatomically and mechanically correct will create optimum power output and should look like the illustration shown in Figure 9-3 (b). This type of pattern enables riders to create an effective force transfer to the pedals as they push down-over the top, finish driving down and forward through the power phase, and allow the recovery leg to clear by pulling the foot/leg back and up at the bottom of the stroke. RealRyder does not encourage actively pulling up the pedal on the recovery phase. Instead, the key with the recovery leg is that it gets "pushed" by the leg that is entering into the power phase but must not interfere with momentum. The cyclist must "unweight" or "unload" the pedal in the recovery phase by pulling up the leg, which effectively "gets the recovery leg out of the way" so that it does not inhibit pedal stroke speed. Chapter 15, *Ryding Skills and Drills*, offers a complementary discussion on this subject.

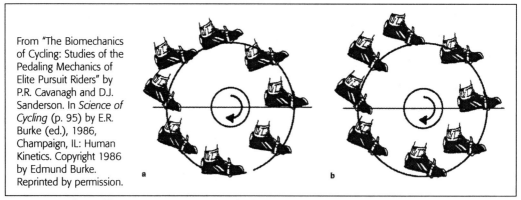

From "The Biomechanics of Cycling: Studies of the Pedaling Mechanics of Elite Pursuit Riders" by P.R. Cavanagh and D.J. Sanderson. In *Science of Cycling* (p. 95) by E.R. Burke (ed.), 1986, Champaign, IL: Human Kinetics. Copyright 1986 by Edmund Burke. Reprinted by permission.

a                    b

Figure 9-3. The ankling pattern recommended in popular bicycling literature (a) and the ankling pattern that Peter Cavanagh and David Sanderson determined that highly successful elite pursuit riders use (b)

# Pedal Technique and Stroke Summary

The pedals are the primary site of energy transfer from the rider to the bike. While both legs are moving in a synchronous motion, they are 180 degrees opposite of each other, which means that when the right leg is pushing down during the power phase, the left leg is in recovery.

Although cyclists move their feet in circles during pedaling, the forces applied to the pedal from the foot are not circular. Many inexperienced riders will pedal by contracting the quadriceps to push down forcefully, rather than forward, during the downstroke and then rest on the upstroke, rather than unweighting or unloading the pedal. Riders should not attempt to lift the pedal up, but rather lift the leg up and "stay ahead of the recovery pedal," eliminating any interference of pedal speed. An inappropriate pedaling style can hinder the power contributions of other muscle groups in the legs, calves, and hamstrings, and can destroy the synergy that represents optimal pedaling economy. Furthermore, *only* pushing down on the pedals creates a short, uneven revolution and limits the momentum of the pedal stroke with each revolution.

***Optimal pedal stroke…***A more efficient pedal stroke is adopted by experienced cyclists who *pull-back* as they ride through the beginning of the upstroke (i.e., recovery phase). It should be noted that this action is not the same as simply pulling the pedal up. However, if riders pull *back* starting at the 5 to 6 o'clock portion of the stroke to about the 7 o'clock position, more force is applied across the bottom of the down stroke. More force application results from the lower-leg muscles contributing to the motion, thereby making it possible to apply power for a longer period in the upstroke. This action creates a smooth transition from the upstroke to the down stroke. The pulling-back technique is a skill that requires practice to develop and can result in a fluid, more powerful pedal stroke.

Maintaining proper body position is especially important to the stroke when the cyclist moves from a seated to a standing position. Pedaling form and optimal technique are greatly influenced by bike set-up, proper load and cadence.

# Physiology of Cycling Primer

When a cyclist starts a training session, the body responds immediately to ensure that the circulating oxygen, nutrients (carbohydrates, proteins, and fats), hormones and byproducts are delivered and/or eliminated at an increased rate. To this end, several changes occur in the body's cardiovascular system.

❏ *Heart rate and cardiac output.* A cyclist on the move experiences an increase in *heart rate* (HR), which is measured in beats per minute (bpm). In addition, the amount of blood pumped from the heart each time it beats also increases, a factor that is referred to as *stroke volume* (SV). These two variables, HR and SV, represent *cardiac output.* A measure of how well the heart is performing its function of moving the blood through the body, cardiac output is the volume of blood pumped by the heart in one minute, a measure that is equal to SV multiplied by HR.

❑ *Respiration.* A person's breathing rate is also affected when aerobic exercise is initiated. The *sympathetic nervous system* stimulates the respiratory muscles to increase the rate of breathing. Metabolic byproducts, such as *lactate* and carbon dioxide, stimulate the brain to bring about an increase in respiration. Furthermore, higher *systolic blood pressure,* caused by the increased force of each heartbeat and by the elevated cardiac output, opens blood flow to additional *alveoli* in the lungs, which increases the exerciser's rate of breathing and allows more oxygen to enter the blood.

❑ *Fat utilization.* Perhaps one of the most important benefits of engaging in aerobic training on a regular basis is that it enhances the body's ability to use fat as fuel during exercise, a factor that ultimately helps class participants lose weight. Proper training also leads to an improvement in the ability of certain enzymes to release fat from *adipose tissue,* which allows the fat to be used as a substance to drive aerobic metabolism during exercise. This increased reliance on fat for fuel enables the muscles to conserve their limited supplies of carbohydrate *(glycogen)* and produce less lactate, which allows the exerciser to work at higher intensities for longer periods of time before getting fatigued. Lactate is a substance produced during intense effort. If it accumulates in the muscle tissue, it is a sign that energy is being used faster than it can be produced aerobically. Too much lactate interferes with the muscle's ability to contract and causes labored breathing, fatigue, and a discomfort, which is sometimes described as a "burning" sensation. A well-planned aerobic exercise program can actually result in a cyclist developing an increased tolerance to the lactate produced during intense exercise. As a result, the rider's level of cardiovascular endurance and work output is enhanced.

❑ *Fiber type.* An important factor that determines a muscle's performance capabilities is its composition of fiber types. Two primary types of skeletal muscle fibers exist: *slow-twitch (type 1) and fast-twitch (type 2) fibers.*

Fast-twitch fibers are large in diameter as a result of densely-packed strands of protein called *myofibrils.* They contain large glycogen reserves and relatively few mitochondria, which are important structures inside cells that are partly responsible for aerobic metabolism. Because the force produced by a muscle fiber is directly proportional to its size, muscles dominated by fast-twitch fibers produce powerful contractions. On the other hand, fast-twitch fibers fatigue relatively rapidly because their contractions use ATP in large amounts. Fast-twitch fiber force production is primarily dependent on anaerobic metabolism.

Slow-twitch muscle fibers are only about half the diameter of fast-twitch fibers and take three times as long to contract after stimulation. Slow-twitch fibers can contract for extended periods. Because slow-twitch fibers contain more mitochondria and an extensive network of tiny blood vessels, they have a dramatically higher oxygen supply. With their oxygen reserves and a more efficient blood supply, the mitochondria of slow-twitch fibers can contribute more ATP during contraction. Slow-twitch fibers are primarily dependent on aerobic metabolism.

Most muscles contain a mixture of fiber types. The percentage of fast-twitch versus slow-twitch fibers in each muscle is genetically determined and varies from one individual to another. These differences influence a person's ability to successfully perform speed and power events versus endurance events, which is a major reason why an individual's athletic capability is strongly influenced by genetics.

❑ *Power output/caloric expenditure.* In endurance and fitness cycling, calorie-burning potential and power output (resistance/cadence/mph/watts) are largely determined by how fit one is and genetics, as related to percentage of fast- or slow-twitch fiber type. In other words, individuals who want to be a world class cyclist should choose their parents well. Fortunately, all riders can improve greatly from their genetic starting point.

## Key Point

*In cycling, as pedal resistance increases while cadence remains constant, power rises. Similarly, if cadence increases while the resistance stays the same, power also increases. If both cadence and resistance increase power output increases.*

❑ *Cycling power.* Power is either the rate at which muscular force is applied to move a load or the rate at which physical work is done. In other words, power is the product of force and speed.

❑ *Class design application.* As a rule, indoor-cycling classes tend to have participants who possess various skill sets and strengths. Some riders, especially those individuals who are strong and can push through higher resistance or "gears," will benefit from improving their endurance. In turn, those riders who are already proficient at maintaining higher cadence and lighter loads can become more powerful by developing the ability to work at higher resistance levels and slower speeds.

A working knowledge of the science and physiology of cycling, along with an understanding of the training approaches that personalize the ride can help to ensure that riders are challenged with the most effective workouts possible (refer to Chapters 10-15).

# 10

# Cadence and Resistance

Aside from the obvious methods of applying resistance (gears) to the flywheel to increase the intensity level on an indoor cycle or pedaling quicker (increasing the cadence) research (Loy, et al., 2009) has shown that the RealRyder bike also allows cyclists to increase their level of exertion through leaning and turning, and increased core activation because of balance and coordination challenges. Side-to-side movement, balance, leaning and steering can influence intensity—just like on a road bike. One benefit of layering these actions on top of the one-dimensional process of pedaling on a fixed stationary bike is that the rider can achieve a higher level of calorie burning within the same timeframe.

*Preferred cadence and resistance.* The level of resistance enables riders to control the pedal stroke. Cueing riders to adopt a "preferred cadence and resistance" can help participants find the proper combination of resistance and cadence for their ability and goal of the ryde. Also, it is important to debunk the myths that "faster is always better" and "indoor cycling must always be intense." What works well for one individual, may not work equally as efficiently for another.

## Key Point

*Riders should be taught all of the possible options concerning pedaling cadence and resistance that matches perfectly to ryde goal and capability.*

## Measuring Cadence

❏ *Music.* Music offers a perfect option for establishing cadence. Music with a steady rhythm can be particularly useful, since it can help riders maintain a steady cadence or level of effort. Some songs are filled with highs and lows and match well with recommended cadence ranges. Beats per minute (bpm), which varies with music style, can run the gamut from 60 to 200 bpm. Classes can be designed around music. The result can be restrictive for some cyclists and entirely motivating and fun for others. Even when music is used to influence tempo and cadence, riders should be encouraged to "ryde free" and find preferred cadence. Ryders can choose to ride on the beat if that rhythm/cadence suits them. More often than not, riding cadence should be based on the RydeProfile and/or preferred cadence. Let music go along for the ryde rather than the other way around!

Cadence based on a song's bpm can be encouraged, but should not be "required." Contrived cadence—cadence that is determined solely by what song is playing—can be too fast, too slow, just right, dangerous, safe, fun, motivating or just not quite right. For example, a class is riding to an 80 bpm song. An instructor might suggest that the riders stay within plus or minus 5 to 10 rpm of the rhythm, rather than mandating that "everyone stay on the beat of the song." The key point is that every indoor cycling instructor should encourage and guide the ryde, which is based on the RydeProfile/"terrain" challenges—not bpm. A song may be perfect for a steep, tough hill climb (70-75 bpm), but the lyrics, vocal quality and energy of a 50 bpm song can be used to help teach a high-speed cadence drill that helps prepare a rider for an 80 rpm climb—if the class is not required to "ride on the beat." Furthermore, a 50 bpm song can be doubled and work well for a 100 rpm effort. The opposite is also true; a 120 bpm song can work perfectly for a slow-cadence climb at 60 rpm.

## Key Point

*Let music motivate, but not dictate how individuals ride.*

❏ *Metronome.* It is relatively easy to set a specific bpm/cadence using an inexpensive metronome. In fact, an entire indoor-cycling class can be taught to a metronome. While a class may have some motivating music playing lightly in the background, the focus is on cadence. The emphasis of cadence drills should be on leg-speed development, a skill that is highly trainable. Pedal stroke technique and cadence drills go hand-in-hand and are desirable to address weekly.

❏ *Instructor visual.* If instructors can hold the bpm of each song and align it with the cadence goals of the class, riders can key in on the teacher and stick to the cadence, even if the student cannot hear it.

❏ *Counting pedal strokes.* Although counting pedal strokes is challenging, it can be done. An optimal situation is to display a large "swimmer's clock" that is easy for all participants to see. Whether using a digital watch or swimmer's clock, the instructor calls out "ready-set-count," and at 10-seconds ends with a "ready-set-stop." The rider multiplies by six the number of times the leg returned to the top of the pedal stroke during the 10-second period to get a projected rpm/cadence per minute. Over time, riders can "guesstimate" their rpm for seated and standing positions within a three to five plus or minus error. Manual counting to determine cadence is cumbersome at best and "impossible" to do out of the saddle.

❏ *Bike computer.* In a perfect world, all indoor bikes would have an onboard computer that measures watt/power output, mph, distance, calories, time and rpm/cadence. Riders are provided with constant and accurate rpm feedback. In addition, the measurement of rpm using a computer does not interrupt the workout focus and is always immediately available.

# Cadence and Resistance Recommendations

❏ ***Cadence on the "flats"–80 to 100 rpm.*** On flat roads, most riders use a cadence that is about 80 to 100 rpm, while seated. Riders tend to move in and out of the saddle to "stretch" or provide a break from the seated position. Moving in and out of the saddle is accomplished by "clicking up a gear," turning the pedals quickly for a few seconds and then sliding smoothly back onto the seat.

**Key Point**

> *If riders insist on using a fast cadence and prioritize pedaling wildly above appropriate resistance/cadence, training will suffer. This holds true whether the primary goal is to lose weight or become a better cyclist. Pedaling fast does not necessarily equate with training effectively.*

Very few riders can maintain pedaling efficiency as rpm moves toward 120. If riders push the extremes they should do so using correct form. "No bouncing in the seat–feel the *heat*." The "heat" riders feel are their legs working to overcome the gear or resistance that has been added.  "No 'free-riding'; no chasing an un-loaded flywheel!"

**Key Point**

> *More trouble than benefit–as it relates to excessive rpm–awaits riders who are less fit and skilled.*

Skilled and fit riders tend to ride using higher rpm when compared to less fit or novice riders for a given work load. Training at a high rpm for improved leg speed/turnover, which represents an important neurological training component, should be limited to leg-speed drills for serious cyclists.

Related closely to riding at a realistic cadence is understanding the importance of controlling "flywheel momentum" by using appropriate resistance. The indoor training focus of riders should be on a preferred cadence that either matches outdoor specificity and/or allows the rider to maintain form, good pedal technique and proper body position.

Cyclists can ride a flat road using a heavy gear and slow cadence (below 80 rpm), but by doing so they will have missed the training focus and benefit of riding a flat road in the recommended cadence range as it relates to pedaling efficiency, leg speed and training effect. It is not wrong, or right, to ride slowly or quickly. Flat road cadence is simply different than what is required for a seated hill or standing climb. Riders and instructors should define what the riding focus is for each ride segment which is largely dictated by body position, gear choice, pedaling cadence and training/performance/conditioning goals. Stick to and create RydeProfile plans so that the same emphasis is not used all the time.

❏ *Cadence on a hill or climb—60 to 80 rpm.* Lance Armstrong can turn a cadence of 100 rpm on an intense climb. An equally impressive Jan Ullrich climbs the same hill at 70 rpm. From novice to very strong riders—including some professionals—a range of 60 to 80 rpm has been shown to be the average and most efficient cadence range. Can a rider climb at 80 to 90 rpm? Of course! If a climbing style, and for that matter any riding style, suits a rider's physical characteristics, it is never a matter of right or wrong, but more a degree of appropriateness as it relates to each person's individual makeup.

For an individual who asks if he/she can tackle a climb with quicker turnover, the appropriate question to toss right back is, "I don't know, can you?" If the rider can maintain the desired power output (rpm and gear) and good riding form the answer is, "Yes!" Cycling can be very personal, which is why everyone at RealRyder likes to RydeReal.

❏ *Slow standing recovery cadence.* Many riders love a slow, standing recovery at about 60 rpm. Riders do not always have to work hard when out of the saddle. A standing effort can range from recovery, to moderate and somewhat sustainable, to all-out exhaustive and of short duration. In any of these situations having an appropriate level of resistance is the key. Riders should always have resistance/gear or "feel the road," whenever they are out of the saddle. Standing is not fun and totally ineffective without proper resistance. A slow recovery stand—maybe it occurs at the end of a ride or after riders have busted their legs over the top of a tough hill or have pushed a sustained seated flat road ride—can feel very good. How should it be done? Add enough resistance to slow cadence to about 60 rpm while maintaining a smooth pedal stroke and stay balanced over the pedals/bottom bracket. Do not move forward onto the bars or mash through or "bounce off" the bottom of the stroke.

# Cadence and Resistance:
# Part art (experience), part science!

Cadence recommendations are based on years of research that have examined optimal ranges for every imaginable riding variation (lactate threshold, hills, flats, sprints) and body type ($VO_2$max, fiber type, training history). Resistance/gear choice directly influences cadence and vice versa, as well as intensity.

*RealRyde cadence.* To discuss either cadence or "gear" without the other is not "real." Also, riders should know that a preferred cadence indoors is usually 10 rpm quicker than a comparable level outdoors, because of the "flywheel effect." Riders must learn to control this "momentum factor" which can be virtually eliminated by using an appropriate level of resistance. Riders should "feel the road" and avoid "chasing the flywheel."

## Key Point

*Resistance builds strong legs. Load drives training effect. Riders always have resistance outdoors. RydeReal!*

While the recommendations of RealRyder Indoor Cycling are grounded in an evidence-based foundation, research is ongoing to continue to narrow the science down concerning the issue. Ultimately, a black-and-white recommendation range will *never* exist, because of the numerous individual physiological, neuro-physiological and biomechanical variables that must be taken into account when comparing performance from rider to rider.

Common cadence recommendations vary from 60 to 120 rpm. Most riders fall in the norms of research based ranges that provide an effective and safe framework from which to ride.

***RealLife cadence scenario***...The following real-life cadence scenario—which compares two elite riders—is an excellent starting point to fully understand why a black and white cadence recommendation does not exist.

During Lance Armstrong's electrifying 2001 Tour de France ascent of Alpe D'Huez—8% mean grade; 14-km climb; 38 minutes long; near maximal effort at 475-500 watts; average speed was 22 kph, or > 12 mph; mean cadence was 100 rpm; using a 39 x 23 gear—his superiority speaks for itself. Needless to say, he got the job done. On the same ascent, Jan Ullrich used a more common pedaling rpm of 70, average speed 21 kph and a 41 x 17 gear. He did not get the job done.

First, a counter to anyone who might argue, "Why should I not consider climbing hills faster than 80 rpm? Lance does it!" The hard and fast answer: "The questioner is not Lance!" In turn, someone might pose the following question, "Is Armstrong's approach—it is on the fringe of extreme with regard to pedaling cadence on flats and climbs—optimal or to be strived for whether you are an elite cyclist or a fitness enthusiast? The answer is no and yes, but probably not.

## Key Point

*Pedal cadence and resistance (gear) choices are only as good as they match up to rider capability.*

Another tour rider, Bjarne Riijs, won the Tour de France in 1996 and had a similar astonishing ride during an ascent of Hautacam. His approach was entirely differently than Armstrong's. His pedaling cadence was 70 rpm or less, and he used the front chain ring for the climb, which was a 53-tooth ring. Armstrong used a 39-tooth ring to accomplish his feat. Indeed, both "got it done" using very different pedaling styles.

## Key Point

*Cadence is best evaluated from a perspective of whether or not the rider can maintain riding efficiency and form. Preferred cadence must match-up to the rider's physical traits, capability/skill and current level of fitness.*

***Final thought***...If riders were hammering an 8 to 9 percent grade climb (very steep), most would not be pedaling 12 mph at 90 to 100 rpm. Think Armstrong! Instead, they would be looking down at their back cog set—hoping that maybe, just maybe, they had another gear left. They would look again a few minutes later and curse themselves for not buying that compact chainring set! Very good cyclists can suffer and put up astonishing performance numbers. Some can drop to 50 rpm, "mashing and weaving like hell," just to survive and keep the bike moving.

## Key Point

*In cycling, exceptions always exist to the rules.*

At RealRyder we love the pureness and individuality of our sport—which is why the opportunity to ride outdoors, while indoors—has been a primary focus since day one. RydeReal!

# 11

# Gauging Effort Level: RPE and HR

The most effective way to measure and monitor cardiorespiratory effort involves blending real-data measurement (heart rate) with subjective judgment (rating exertion). This blend is used to determine appropriate exercise intensity and to gauge fitness improvements. Rating perceived exertion (RPE), heart rate (HR) and lactate threshold (LT) are all part of the mix. Lactate threshold heart rate (LTHR) training focuses on a more sophisticated and useful approach to measure intensity (Chapter 12, *Energy Zone Training*). The information presented in this chapter provides a review and update on how to effectively use RPE and HR.

**Key Point**

*Chapter 12,* Energy Zone Training, *explains the science behind the use of LTHR and "why" LTHR training is the preferred method when compared to training at a percentage of MaxHR.*

## Gauging Exercise Intensity

What is the value in measuring exercise intensity? Knowing the appropriate "training-sensitive zone" allows riders to ride at a level that improves conditioning, maximizes time usage and results—and keeps HR/RPE in an appropriate range.

❑ *Methods for monitoring exercise intensity.* Numerous methods exist for monitoring exercise intensity. Many coaches and trainers use one or more of five common methods.

1. Percentage of maximal heart rate (maxHR)

   a. MaxHR is predicted by using a formula based on age-related norms (220-age). Training ranges are calculated by multiplying the estimated maxHR by two percentages (e.g., 50% and 85%) or "two target HRs"—to establish the training range, which is based on a percentage of maxHR.

2. Heart rate maximum reserve (HRR)

   a. HRR (heart rate reserve), based on Karvonen's formula, is also used to estimate an intensity level or training range. Many health/fitness and sports medicine professionals prefer HRR over maxHR. Though similar to a percentage of maximal heart rate, training at a percentage of HRR takes into account the rider's resting heart rate (RHR), but still has the same inherent limitations when compared to training at a percentage of maxHR.

3. Rating of perceived exertion (RPE)

   a. RPE uses perception of effort. We recommend that RPE be gauged using a zero to ten numerical rating scale and verbal exertion cues—such as easy or moderate—that coincide with the numerical rating and how the rider perceives the effort (Chapter 12, *Energy Zone Training.*)

4. Talk test

   a. The talk test, a general measure of a person's level of breathlessness, is often used in combination with RPE.

5. Preferred exertion (PE)

   a. This measure involves having the exerciser choose a "preferred" exertion level, often in combination with RPE.

*Note:* The first two methods for monitoring exercise intensity are used to estimate either a target heart rate (THR) or a training heart rate range (THRR). A THRR is calculated when two THRs are determined by multiplying maxHR or HRR by two different percentages (e.g., 70% and 75%).

**Key Point**

*At RealRyder a combination of working at a percentage of LTHR and using RPE is preferred for monitoring exercise intensity. Refer to Chapter 12.*

# Training-Sensitive Zone Primer

The training-sensitive zone has its physiological basis in the laboratory. Heart rate (HR) is the number of heartbeats that occurs within a specified timeframe. Maximal aerobic capacity ($VO_2$max), defined as an individual's maximum capacity to generate adenosine triphosphate (ATP or energy) 'aerobically,' improves if exercise is intense enough to increase heart rate to about 70 percent of maxHR. This level is equivalent to about 50 to 55 percent of $VO_2$max or HRR. This degree of effort appears to be the *minimal* stimulus required for training improvements in *maximal* aerobic capacity, though frequency and duration also have an impact on this factor. This level of effort is not necessary, however, to achieve health-related goals. For deconditioned individuals, the training threshold may be closer to 60 percent of maxHR, which corresponds to about 40 to 45 percent of $VO_2$max. The lower limits for a training-sensitive threshold related to improved aerobic capacity (but not necessarily improved $VO_2$max) depend on a rider's current fitness capacity.

## Key Point

*Seemingly minimal efforts should be encouraged. Work efforts that take riders beyond what they are accustomed to can contribute significantly to positive conditioning effects and health gains.*

# HRR and VO$_2$

For nearly all levels of submaximal exercise, the percentage of maxHR does not equal the same percentage of $VO_2$max or aerobic capacity. On the other hand, the Karvonen formula, which is reviewed in greater detail later in this chapter, is used to predict HRR and correlates directly to $VO_2$max. Figure 11-1 illustrates the relationship between percent max$VO_2$ and percent max heart rate.

**Relation Between Percent Max VO$_2$ and Percent Max Heart Rate**

| % Max HR | HRR or % Max VO$_2$ |
|----------|---------------------|
| 50 | 28 |
| 60 | 42 |
| 70 | 56 |
| 80 | 70 |
| 90 | 83 |
| 100 | 100 |

From McArdle, W.D., F.I. Katch & V.L. Katch, 1996, *Exercise Physiology: Energy, Nutrition and Human Performance*, 4th edition. Baltimore, MD: Williams & Wilkins. Table 21.6, p. 403. Reprinted with permission.

Figure 11-1. The relationship between percent maxVO$_2$ and percent max heart rate

# Accuracy of Predicting THRR

Prediction equations (e.g., involving 220-age) that are used to estimate maxHR and from which training or target heart rates are derived have a large amount of error inherent to them. Error ranges from plus or minus 10 to 12 beats per minute, with second and third standard deviations as high as plus or minus 20 beats in either direction from the mean/average. For example, for a 40 year old the mean/average maxHR would be 180 (220-40=180). But, the true maxHR could range from 160 to 200.

Understanding each of the variables that can affect the accuracy of HR training can provide insight into the capabilities of whether or not a predicted THRR that is based on a maxHR can accurately reflect exercise intensity. The beauty of LTHR training is that a maxHR is not required.

# When Heart Rate Monitoring
# May Not Be the Best Choice

Using heart rate may not be the best option to monitor exercise intensity for the following groups:

❏ People taking medication that can slow, or otherwise affect their HR. If HR is used, the exercising HR must be determined while the individual is medicated (i.e., taking any prescribed medication) and under medical supervision, so that the heart rate is more likely to reflect the actual effort of the exercising participant.

❏ Participants who are unable to accurately monitor their HR. In this instance, the accuracy of the riders' pulse counts or of the heart rate monitor they are using must be checked.

❏ Individuals, such as those in cardiac rehabilitation, who require very accurate heart rate monitoring.

Mounting evidence continues to indicate that RPE may be a better choice to gauge exercise intensity, in some instances, in terms of effectiveness and safety. To use RPE most effectively, the relationship between heart rate (cardiac response) and RPE (physiological response) has to be accurately established. Creating this relationship simply involves assigning an RPE to various workloads/efforts and then matching the actual HR response to the perception of effort. In time, riders can "guess" their riding HR within + or −5 beats per minute.

**Key Point**

*At RealRyder, we believe that using both RPE and heart rate is the best approach, especially when HR is used in conjunction with working at a percentage of LTHR.*

# Has Heart Rate Monitoring Been Overemphasized?

Many professionals believe that THR has been overemphasized for average exercise participants and can, in many instances, lead to inappropriate exercise intensities—a situation that includes exercising too hard, as well as exercising with too little effort. The effects can be quite negative and contribute to injury, a lack of results for the time invested and exercise dropout.

Monitoring exercise heart rate precisely and accurately is probably of greatest importance to competitive athletes and cardiac patients. For example, high-intensity interval training for highly conditioned athletes is very precise. Both the effort and recovery of the interval are closely monitored in the belief that this manipulation will produce optimal training results and accomplish specific "energy system training." Chapter 12 provides more information on training a percentage of LTHR.

**Key Point**

*Riders should be taught how to "tune-in" to their bodies. Using a combination of heart rate monitoring and RPE—produce the safest, most effective and time efficient result.*

# Rating Exertion

An easy and practical way to monitor effort is based on a rating of perceived exertion (RPE) or "perception of effort." Getting in tune with this "sense" allows riders to "check in" with how they are feeling at any given moment. When subjective judgment is used in conjunction with HR monitoring a double check on accuracy and effectiveness is provided.

***RPE scale***...RPE can be taught by associating HR response with a particular numerical rating and its assigned descriptive terms on a scale of 1 to 10. For example, an easy-to-moderate level of effort could be rated 2 to 3 numerically and "somewhat easy" to "moderate" descriptively. Chapter 12, *Energy Zone Training*, provides detail on this subject and an RPE 0-10 Exertion Scale for reference.

# RPE and Improved Fitness

When riders become better conditioned, their perception of exertion at a given level of effort will feel easier. To attain the same RPE, workload must be increased. Equally true is that as fitness levels increase, the intensity of activity must increase if continued improvements are desired. Each rider's individual training situation and goals should determine that person's training intensity level.

**Key Point**

*Ultimately, all riders should take personal responsibility for working at a level of intensity that they perceive as reasonable but challenging.*

# Phases of an Indoor Cycling Workout

This section provides a primer on the phases of an indoor cycling workout. Additional information on this subject is presented in Chapter 14, *Creating a Ryde—Planning Your Class Workouts.*

❏ *Warm-Up*

A warm-up immediately prior to physical activity provides the body with a period of adjustment, moving from rest to exercise. A properly designed warm-up improves performance and decreases the chance of injury by preparing the individual mentally and physically for activity. In a group-cycling class, the warm-up "build" should last between five to ten minutes, and if structured correctly, participants will not realize when the warm-up transitions into the ride. The cycling warm-up should be intense enough to increase the body's core temperature and cause some sweating, but not so intense as to cause fatigue. Typically, riders should pedal at a comfortable pace and use light resistance so that they familiarize themselves with the bike and prepare their bodies for the demands of the workout.

❏ *Conditioning Phase*

The intensity and duration of cardiovascular exercise ultimately determine the health or fitness outcome for the exerciser.

As a general rule, everyone can progress to working slightly out of their "comfort zone" for portions of the ride. Advanced riders may be able to tolerate longer-duration classes (45 to 60 minutes) following a RydeProfile that incorporates high-intensity challenges into the workout. More often than not, an instructor will have to manage a variety of fitness levels in an indoor cycling class. The appropriate intensity for cardiovascular exercise depends on several factors, including the exerciser's level of conditioning and that person's fitness goals.

It is also important to remember that overweight or deconditioned people reach their cardiovascular capacity more quickly and with less effort. The opposite is true for fit riders.

❏ *Cool-Down*

The cool-down provides the rider's body with a period of adjustment—that moves from exercise to rest—and may be defined as low-intensity riding performed immediately after the conditioning phase of a workout. In a cycling class, an appropriate cool-down is five to ten minutes in length, performed at a light resistance, and continues until the heart rate and breathing rate return closer to the resting state. The main objective of a cool-down is to facilitate recovery and allow the cardiovascular system to return to a lowered level of demand. Mobility and/or stabilization training may be incorporated immediately after the cool-down period.

# 12

# Energy Zone (EZ) Training

Energy zone (EZ) training is very important to help develop "speed" and power output—in addition to increased caloric expenditure and fitness gains. Planned properly, a deep sense of accomplishment comes with new found riding ability and endurance. Precise guidance as to how hard one should work—and how the rider gets there focusing on pedal cadence and resistance—is essential.

**Key Point**

*Energy Zone Training defines "why" lactate threshold heart rate (LTHR) training is the preferred method to measure effort when using heart rate.*

To monitor level of effort effectively use RPE (rating perceived exertion) and heart rate (HR). Every rider should also be familiar with lactate threshold (LT)—independent of fitness level. All three can be used to ensure that the cardiovascular system is completely trained by using a variety of work efforts that have purpose. The key to monitoring effort is to identify how the intensity feels at various levels of output (Figures 12-1 and 12-2).

**Key Point**

*Effective intensity monitoring is based on understanding how the effort should feel and tuning into LTHR!*

# Establishing Energy Training Zones Primer

EZ Training makes coaching "intensity" fun, simple and effective! Also, refer to Chapter 13, *Coaching a Ryde.*

*Understanding lactate threshold (LT)…*Based on the predominant type of energy metabolism—which is dependent on intensity of effort and fitness level—two types of thresholds can be differentiated. The aerobic threshold (AerT) represents the limit of *predominantly* aerobic metabolism, where sufficient oxygen is present to metabolize carbohydrates and fats with little lactate accumulation (e.g., < 2 mmol/L of lactate). Lactate threshold (LT)—*sometimes referred to as ventilatory breaking point, AT or anaerobic threshold, OBLA (onset of blood lactic acid)*—is where the upper limit of lactate equilibrium occurs, meaning lactate build up and breakdown are balanced with no significant accumulation of lactate occurring. This generally occurs at 4 mmol/L of lactate in the blood. The dominant energy substrate utilized at LT is carbohydrate and it is metabolized through aerobic and anaerobic energy pathways. Fit trainees can reach 60%-65% of maximum oxygen uptake (maxVO$_2$) at AerT and 85%-95% at LT. Unfit riders can only reach 45%-50% of maximum oxygen uptake (maxVO$_2$) at AerT and 50%-70% at LT.

*Note:* RealRyder Indoor Cycling does not distinguish between AT, LT, OBLA and ventilatory breaking point. We prefer to cite LT and LTHR, rather than AT or other similar physiological reference points.

# Energy Zone (EZ) Training

### If training zones are established referencing a percentage of LTHR—five exact training zones can be established (Carmichael 2009):

I.  Recovery, warm-up and cool-down level of effort.

II. a. 50%-91% of LTHR field test (RPE 4-5)—Endurance/"cruising" phase that challenges aerobic tempo; effort can be sustained using predominantly aerobic energy production.
    *Note:* a fit athlete can ride at LT (91%) for long periods and rate it as "cruising."

    b. 88%-91% of LTHR field test (RPE 5-6)—Challenging aerobic tempo.

III. 92%-94% of LTHR field test (RPE 7-8)—Challenging LT work.

IV. 95%-97% of LTHR field test (RPE 7-9)—Climbing/seated interval repeat that increases power at LT.

V. 100% of Maximum (RPE 10)—Increased power at VO2max; true "all out" sprints and intervals are the only efforts that reach an RPE of 10.

**Reference:** (Carmichael 2009), pgs. 82; 86-87

***If training zones are established referencing a <u>percentage of maxHRR</u>—based on research—four broad training zones can be established:***

I.  50%-70% of best performance/maxHRR (RPE 2-5)—Recovery/regenerative stage

II.  70%-85% of best performance/maxHRR (RPE 5-8)—Foundational endurance stage

III. 80%-90% of best performance/maxHRR (RPE 7-8)—Development stage

IV. 90% of best performance/maxHRR (RPE 9-10)—Competition/power stage

# Monitoring Intensity

Helping students estimate, control and monitor intensity level is an important aspect of the *RealRyder Indoor Cycling Program.*

***Why RPE?*** It would not be logical that everyone in class could climb a hill using the same resistance and cadence. However, ALL riders can feel the road begin to turn upward under them or steepen. ALL can increase to a 2-3 RPE, while holding different cadences and using different gears. A rider's RPE 8 might be another's 6. It is possible classes will have a whole range of riders from novice to pro. Using RPE allows everyone to work at a level of effort (resistance, cadence) and body position (seated or standing) that matches to current skill and fitness levels. Using RPE can help to motivate and challenge anyone at their current fitness level even though the class has a wide range of competency. This scenario represents the beauty of RPE! Cue resistance or intensity changes by referring to Figures 12-1 and 12-2.

RPE is best used in conjunction with HR monitoring and the opposite holds true as well. When used together, HR and RPE create the most effective approach. If forced to choose between HR and RPE, RPE would win. It is that valuable! However, the greatest synergy exists when using both to monitor intensity and as a "checks and balance" to ensure that both feedback tools are providing accurate information.

## 5Ts Relate Directly to Intensity and Effort Level

1.  ***Teach cadence with a metronome, manually, music or a computer.***

2.  ***Teach with RPE/LTHR.***

3.  ***Teach proper resistance/gear.***

4.  ***Teach power (resistance/cadence combination).***

5.  ***Teach ALL riders to associate with lactate threshold (LT).***

| Energy Zone Training RPE 0-10 Exertion Scale/Percentage of LTHR and Max Effort | | |
|---|---|---|
| **CV/Aerobic Training** | **Numerical Rating** | **Exertion Cues** |
| Rest | 0-1 | Very easy |
| I. Recovery, Warm-Up, Cool Down; Easy to Moderate Steady State | 2-3 | Easy to moderate |
| II. Endurance/Aerobic Tempo | 4-5 50%-91% of LTHR | Moderate to hard; sustainable |
| Endurance/Aerobic Tempo | 5-6 88%-91% of LTHR | Challenging; effort can be sustained |
| III. Lactate Threshold | 7-8 92%-94% of LTHR | More challenging LT work; sustainable; below LT; starting to push "limits" |
| IV. Power At Lactate Threshold | 7-9 95%-97% of LTHR | Effort increases power at LT; not "all out"; very challenging; below LT |
| V. Anaerobic Power Interval | 10 100% of Max Effort | Very hard sprint or interval training; "all out"; above LT |

*Note:* Multiply LTHR by the upper and lower limits of the suggested range in each zone to establish upper and lower training range limits.

Figure 12-1. RPE 0-10 Exertion Scale/Percentage of LTHR and Max Effort

| Energy Zone Training RPE 0-10 Exertion Scale/Percentage of MaxHRR | | | |
|---|---|---|---|
| **Level** | **% maxVO$_2$/% max/HRR** | **Training Adaptations** | **Type of Training** |
| I (RPE 2-3) (easy to moderate) | 50-70 (50-60%; LTs of untrained occur here) | Aerobic energy sources/ pathways developed | Over distance/ endurance training |
| II (RPE 2-3) (moderate plus) | 65-75 (common intensity; too much focus?) | Capillary, mitochondria development; fatty acid utilization | Endurance foundation/ base training |
| III (RPE 4-5) (somewhat hard to challenging) | 70-80 (common intensity; too much focus?) | FOG fibers, glycolysis, O$_2$ transport; training improvements | Endurance foundation/ base training |
| IV (RPE 6-8) (challenging to hard) | 75-90 (most trained LTs occur between 80-90%) | FOG, AT/LT, O$_2$ transport; lactate clearance training and improvement | Interval and race pace training; improve LT threshold |
| V (RPE 9-10) (all out to very hard) | 90-100 (peak intensities) | FT, FG, speed, neural adaptation, muscle coordination | Improve max VO$_2$; racing; peaking; economy/efficiency |

*Note:* Multiply maxHRR by the upper and lower limits of the suggested range in each zone to establish upper and lower training range limits.

Figure 12-2. Energy Zone (EZ) Training using a percentage of maxHRR as a reference

# Training at a Percentage of
# Lactate Threshold Heart Rate (LTHR)

The *Energy Zone Training* figures (12-1, LTHR; 12-2, maxHRR) use a percentage of LTHR or maxHRR to calculate training zones. Training at a percentage of maxHRR is illustrated because this methodology is familiar and common. We recognize that many instructors and programs will continue to use a percentage of maxHRR or maxHR to gauge training effort. Why then, a discussion on training at a percentage of LTHR?

**Key Point**

*Welcome to New School and LTHR Training!*

Though LT training for serious athletes is not new—and because calculating training ranges from a maxHRR is so ingrained in the fitness industry—LTHR training is considered somewhat "radical," simply because it is different.

**Key Point**

*Teach all riders how LT feels! Training at a percentage of LTHR is easy and effective!*

*Lactate threshold (LT) and what it feels like...* LT—challenging but breathing can still be controlled—is critical for ALL riders to associate with for effective and safe training. LT is a rallying point that ALL training should revolve around. Riders can train at, just below, well below or above LT.

**Key Point**

*Everyone must come to know LT. LT pops up when a rider pushes an RPE of 7-9 and he/she is working at 92 to 97 percent of LTHR.*

LT feels somewhat like you are starting to push your limits. At the point you are challenged (RPE 7-9)—but can maintain the effort—is where LT occurs.

# Establishing Lactate Threshold

The lactate threshold reference point is easy to pinpoint using a field test.

*LTHR field test…* A field test consists of an *average* HR calculation of 1) *several* efforts (e.g., two 15 or 8 minute bouts) or 2) a *sustained* effort over 20 to 30 minutes. The effort, regardless of length of test chosen, should reflect the highest speed/rpm/power output that can be sustained over the test duration. LTHR field tests challenge participants but provide objective data about LT. In turn, this personalized data provides everyone who uses LTHR an opportunity to train smarter and improve performance.

*Note:* Use a wireless HR monitor that calculates average HR (avgHR) over the specific test duration when establishing LTHR. Even if a HR monitor is used that can provide an avgHR it is a good idea to record HR at every minute for the test duration. Recording 1-minute HRs allows riders who do not have the "avgHR" feature to calculate avgHR by dividing the sum of 1-minute HRs by the number of minutes the rider was tested. It is also useful for some riders/coaches to analyze the 1-minute interval HR responses. A useable LTHR reference is simple to establish using two 8 minute tests.

*Test protocol…* For each 8 minute test the protocol requires a warm-up, a suggested ride cadence of 80 to 90 rpm to keep power output high, attaining top "speed" about a minute into the test—as well as an effort that can "barely" be maintained for the test length (challenging but you should be able to maintain breath control), and cool down that is about 10-minutes of recovery riding and hydration. Repeat this procedure for the second test.

*Note:* If riders are trading off testing/motivating one another—rather than an instructor testing the entire group simultaneously—the warm-up/test duration for the new person being tested serves as the recovery period. Simply, after a rider finishes a test segment he/she actively recovers off the bike as the other rider preps. It is important to maintain consistency with regard to the exact testing protocol used for reasons related to test validity. If the testing procedure is random the results have less value when one test is compared to another over time.

Riders should put the second test out of mind during the first test and force the pace for the entire test ride. An average HR is calculated for each test. Use the higher of the two average HRs when establishing percentage LTHR training ranges. Join the RealRyder Team for an in-depth LTHR experience at a live workshop or certification.

*Note:* To estimate maxHR divide the avgLTHR by .85; for example, if the field test resulted in an average HR of 175 (LTHR), divide 175 by .85 = 206 (estimated maxHR). This data can be useful to some riders/coaches, but if training using LTHR do NOT use this maxHR estimate to calculate LTHR training ranges.

**Key Point**

*A field test (more precise)—or simply a perception of where riding becomes difficult—can be used to establish the LT reference point.*

*Re-testing...*Retest every 4 to 8 weeks. As riders become fit testing can be done less often. It is likely that LTHR will increase after progressive training (up to a point), which means maxHR will, in theory, go up. Truth lies in the following. MaxHR did not go up; it always existed! LT increased, so it is possible to work at a higher percentage of an individual's maxHR or current LT ceiling!

*Final thought...*In a sense, maxHR is not significant to the training equation. Referencing LTHR and basing workout zones on LTHR is the key to results. Monitoring improvement and planning workouts using LTHR is simple. LTHR training keeps programs "results oriented" and relative at a personal level.

# 13

# Coaching a Ryde

Coaching a ride successfully is based largely on experience, education and intuition. Before moving down the road too far, remember to keep information at each rider's "immediate need" level. When coaching a ride, provide enough "need-to-know" information so that at any point during the ride the following three questions can be answered that are related to 1) What is next? 2) How hard should I be working? and 3) How long do I need to ride hard?

**Key Point**

*Instructors should know their riders and riders should know their bike.*

## First-Time Riders

Coaching a ride and setting a rider up for initial and continued success, at its simplest level, involve the following steps (also see Chapter 6, *RydeRecipe*):

1.  Establish proper bike fit and orient the rider to the bike movement.

2.  Instruct the rider to keep the head, neck, and upper body relaxed and quiet (still)—and "look up the road."

3.  Instruct the rider to pedal a smooth, circular stroke—focusing on a constant transfer of power to the flywheel, via the crank arms/pedals.

4.  Sequence mantra…not too long out of the saddle, add enough resistance in both seated and standing positions; do not be afraid to spend considerable time seated.

5. Riding form mantra…keep weight over the pedals and the hands light on the bars whether seated or standing.

# Know Your Riders

What is the foundation of coaching and instructing?

- Know your craft.
- Know your bike.
- Know your athlete.

**Key Point**

*Coaching is comparable to riding a bike. It is hard to put into words…"Just ride it (e.g., the bike)? There's more to it than that. At some point, however; the essence of the situation is to just ride—after instructors teach, motivate and understand to whom they are teaching."*

# Basic Types of Class Participants

1. Skilled road cyclists and coordinated* cyclists. Fit or unfit, it does not matter. These individuals love the ride and have no learning curve.

2. Uncoordinated* cyclists. These participants tend to be fit and are usually people who ride or teach indoors, but have never been taught to ride correctly.

3. Uncoordinated* cyclists, who tend to be unfit.

*Coordinated (highly skilled) in this context refers to the individual as it relates to handling a bike.*

**Key Point**

*Coordinated people do fine on the RealRyder bike. Fit or unfit—they quickly adapt to the bike movement and ride away into the sunset.*

❏ *Uncoordinated people who are fit enough, will usually figure it out.* Indoor cycling instructors are often concerned for less-fit students, because they may not yet be riding properly. On the other hand, they can still manage to "look okay" while riding because they tend to be very fit. Fit instructors are usually strong enough to muscle the bike into submission. By simply overpowering the bike's reaction to pedal input they are able to stay "on top of the bike" and "hold it in place." They are thinking, "This is awesome, but it's really hard—my students aren't going to be able to do this! "

Therein lies part of the problem. As with many athletic activities, fit people seem to learn more quickly—when, in fact—they are simply strong enough to "fake it," at least better than unfit people can. Only when fatigue starts to set in, will the fit instructor start to figure out a more efficient way to perform the exercise. Eventually, they "get it." Instead of pedaling like they always have and doing a sustained isometric clamp-down on the handlebars, they "learn" that by pedaling smoother and keeping their hips over the front of the saddle and pedals, the bike moves less. These fit-types still have a huge advantage over the unfit individuals, since they get to experience the fun of riding the bike. As a result, they feel like they have accomplished something strenuous. Over time, they gradually begin to feel how they might otherwise control the bike (usually as they begin to fatigue). In turn, the transition from riding inefficiently to properly is gratifying. Basically, they are strong enough to get by until they develop the necessary coordination and skill to perform the ride without unduly exerting themselves. Still, this instructor type often struggle with the "coaching element," because their first instinct is to coach people to do it like they did it (a common attribute of coaches in almost all sports). This approach only works if student-riders are fit enough to struggle (muscle) through the process, can later describe this experience as "fun," and after all of that, still come back and want to ride again. Many instructors and students fall into this category.

❑ *Uncoordinated, unfit people need special treatment and attention.* Not surprisingly, all indoor-cycling instructors want their students to love riding and to quickly absorb whatever they need to in order to become proficient.

If an instructor is teaching novice and unfit participants it is important to encourage students to *play* with bike frame movement. Participants should first, while seated, ride it quietly, then let it get a little loose, and finally, find a happy medium that is their rhythm. While standing, they should honor the smooth pedal stroke, keep their upper body and head quiet, look up the road, feel the bike reacting to their pedaling, try to control it completely, and then let it get a little loose. Finally, they should find their standing rhythm and stabilize the bike's movement with good body position. The participants have transitioned to riding and importantly, are thinking like a pro. Practice, repetition and coaching that reinforce proper ride technique will take care of the rest.

The aforementioned introduction to riding takes five minutes. Hypothetically, the #1s are grinning like "idiots." The #2s are trying desperately to keep up, veins bulging and grimacing mightily. They are on their way to "getting it," and they will be easy to help.

Some of the #3s, however, are looking at their "me-the-coach" like something is wrong with their bike, and are wondering where the old bikes went—the ones that do not wiggle.

Most cycling classes only have a few #3s. Fortunately, instructors who are willing to take their time, be patient and go slowly—can teach anyone. The key to coaching #3s is to teach them to become comfortable staying in the saddle, maintain proper body position, sequence time that is shorter when out of the saddle and insist on correct form. In other words, coaches should encourage #3s to return to the saddle frequently, use enough resistance when standing, keep their weight back over the seat/pedals, and "stay light on the bars." Particularly in a group environment, the #3's can suffer if they are not guided gently. Though instructors should not lose sight of their presence in the classroom—nor should they overwhelm them with correction (attention). But, let them know you've got them!

## Key Point

*With regard to the #3s, a paradox exists. While the #3s are a coach's biggest challenge and biggest reward, they also, ironically, can become a coach's biggest advocate and a virtual word-of-mouth marketing machine—because they will have gained the greatest.*

# Coaching a Ryde

Every cycling instructor/coaching style is unique. Coaching is both a science and art form. The best instructors allow their own excitement about fitness and riding, and their own personality characteristics to come through via their teaching. They understand the importance of not only teaching accurate riding technique, but also the need to model great form or "souplesse."

Experienced coaches can motivate a participant using visual cueing, verbal coaching cues, cycling language, a well thought out RydeProfile (Chapter 14, *Creating a Ryde*), and music to move beyond any real or self-imposed limitation. Seasoned coaches know when to push and when to encourage a rider to hold back. Individualizing and matching the day's workout to each rider's needs/capability is truly an art that is framed within scientific borders.

## Key Point

*Instructors should remember that when coaching a ryde, choreographing a group of riders is not the focus. Instead, they are challenging, encouraging, and motivating cyclists and fitness enthusiasts to improve at a personal level—to achieve individual performance goals.*

# What Makes a Top Indoor-Cycling Coach?

A good indoor cycling coach has a mastery of the topic, knows how to build relationships and recognizes each rider as unique. Qualified coaches:

1.  Are properly trained in cycling biomechanics, physiology, and are able to teach sound cycling technique, form and riding postures.

2.  Teach realistic cadence and resistance (gears) and incorporate heart rate and RPE (rating perceived exertion) into the training sessions.

3.  View themselves as a student, educator and coach.

4.  Never intimidate a class participant into following instructions with loud or otherwise inappropriate behavior.

5.  Correct form breaks, insist on proper bike set-up, and are able to teach on or off the bike.

6.  Offer progressions and regressions, with regard to form, cadence and intensity.

7.  Are able to find the right blend on the intensity continuum—from easy to more challenging, to outright "burn the last match" rides.

8.  Regularly introduce a variety of RydeProfiles and music playlists.

9.  Understand that the class ride is the participant's workout, not the coach's.

10. Identify each rider's goals by communicating with and taking a personal interest in them.

11. Personally acknowledge every rider in each class through eye contact, an encouraging word, a motivational directive, verbal instructional feedback or hands-on communication.

12. Arrange the classroom and bike placement so that the environment is intimate and personal.

13. Are professional, dress appropriately, and are accessible before and after class.

# Know Your Bike

Differences exist between a road bike, the RealRyder indoor cycle and a fixed indoor stationary bike. One cannot teach or ride effectively if it is not clear what the ride can and cannot do and how it reacts to the rider's efforts. While many features of indoor cycles and outdoor bikes are similar, major differences exist (Chapter 4, *RealRyder Indoor Cycle*).

## RydeReal

Individuals who ride outside will appreciate realistic cadence and resistance ranges and everyone can benefit. RydingReal adds a new dimension to any instructor's teaching methodology. Real cycling is never boring. RealRyder is a strong supporter of teaching "real" over "fluff" and "variety for the sake of variety."

❏ *Adding resistance.* It is easy to cue this, for example—by saying "click up a gear," "add a gear," "add two," "pick up a couple," or "pick up a gear," and conversely, "drop a gear," "lose a gear," "drop two," or "drop a couple." Resistance changes can also be guided by using RPE (rating perceived exertion). See Chapter 12, *Energy Zone Training*).

❏ *General cues and teaching.* General cues that encourage and instruct, but don't bully or intimidate, can be used to motivate the group to work harder or easier, or to move out of a personal comfort zone. Riders can slow down their cadence by "adding a gear or two," while maintaining current heart rate. Instructors should cue in advance and set the RydeProfile expectation (e.g., the next six minutes of riding and the task at hand). For example, *"We're going to have three increases in resistance as we climb and crest a moderate hill. Keep your cadence moderate, 80-90 rpms, and stay below lactate threshold. Leave room for three increases, maintain your cadence and don't get to a point of breathlessness."* Scenarios like this help set up a realistic expectation.

*You might coach:*

1. "During the flat road warm up, pedal at 80-85 rpms; keep it light and smooth in the easy blue zone. You're at an RPE of 2-3."

2. "Let's drive this hill seated with a big gear; about 60-70 rpms in the orange, but below threshold. The orange zone is an RPE of 6-8 and we're at the low end."

3. "Guys, we're cresting this climb, but we're staying in the saddle, pushing a heavy gear, 60 rpms; in 30-seconds we'll stand and crank over the top; try to increase your cadence, add a gear and move from low-end orange to high-end orange…pushing above threshold for 10 seconds…out of the saddle optional—let's go!"

4. "It should feel like…"

❏ *Bike flex.* Traditional indoor bikes do not flex or bend. Even road bikes that are placed on stationary trainers do not feel like a real ride. Forced rigidity can be very hard on the bike frame and stressful to the rider's body. Riding this type of set-up doesn't feel right, because the forces of riding are not absorbed or dissipated by the natural movement of the bike, which does not exist on fixed stationary set-ups. A combination of side-to-side bike motion and frame flex achieves this objective out on the road. Outdoors, individuals typically ride with minimal upper-body movement, because excessive motion is simply wasted energy. In outdoor riding, less stress is placed on the body's joints because of the natural motion of the bike moving underneath the rider. More often than not, indoor cycling on stationary fixed bikes actually requires participants to create upper-body motion to compensate for the lack of natural side-to-side movement. While riding the RealRyder cycle, no need exists to compensate for a lack of movement (the flex in the frame and side-side-to movement). That single factor is the essence of RydingReal. Because of the natural side-to-side movement built into the RealRyder cycle, it is not necessary to teach a compensatory technique (e.g., permitting the shoulders of the cyclist to rock side-to-side) that is required on fixed stationary bikes.

❏ *RealRyder cycle fixed-gear and weighted flywheel.* From a teaching/coaching perspective, it is essential to explain to participants that the flywheel creates an inertia that drives the pedals. As a result of the flywheel rotating faster, the pedals also turn over more quickly because of the fixed-gear. This "inertia factor" has huge implications with regard to resistance, cadence selection, and effective riding. When momentum is introduced into the pedal stroke without adequate resistance, the rider can "chase" the flywheel at very high rpms (i.e., 120 to 140) with little effort or power output. In turn, oxygen consumption, calorie burning, and heart-rate response are mitigated, even though the rider's perception of effort (RPE) might be high. The bottom line is that despite spending a lot of time on an indoor fixed stationary bike, riders are not optimizing their potential training results. Riders who fall into this trap will not optimize fitness, weight loss, or progressively achieve their program goals, even though they're investing adequate time cycling. By the same token, they will not become skilled cyclists. Everyone has heard stories about instructors or participants who say they "ride hard" (e.g., ride at a high rpm, with no load/resistance), but still are overweight or at an unacceptable level of fitness. Achieving results is largely defined by power output (resistance and rpm).

## Important Focal Points When Riding a RealRyder Cycle

When riding on a RealRyder bike, the following factors are emphasized, taught and coached:

- Proper riding form, technique and side-to-side movement
- Cadence (Cadence should be realistic.)
- Heart-rate monitoring associated with RPE
- Proper application of resistance (not too much; not too little; turn the knob!)
- Power ("Feel the road!")

❏ *Power output.* Power involves the total amount of work accomplished by the rider. Accordingly, power (work) = speed/velocity (how fast the rider is pedaling or rpms) x load/force (amount of resistance). It is the force or resistance factor that many indoor riders fail to understand. Resistance is a key ingredient that is often missing from indoor classes because of the inertia factor. This factor cannot be emphasized too much. For example, if an individual were to try riding a hill outdoors, or flat road for that matter, it quickly becomes apparent that there is resistance…always.

## Key Point

*While it is hard to eliminate resistance from an outdoor ride—it is relatively easy to do so indoors.*

If cyclists were "spinning" very quickly on the road, but going nowhere fast (in fact, their riding partners were pulling away from them), they would click up a gear to increase their power output in order to keep pace. Indoors, the lack of forward progress (moving down the road) is not as evident. As a result, it is easy to fall into the "inertia trap" or "chasing the flywheel." Even seasoned cyclists might think they are training leg speed (pedal turnover). On the other hand, if their training is not specific to real road riding (e.g., unrealistically fast cadence, with little to no resistance), their efforts will have little practical carryover and minimal impact on their training objectives (e.g., skill development, fitness improvement or weight loss). If the flywheel is driving the pedals and the rider's legs around cyclists will achieve minimal results and the potential for overuse injury increases.

❏ *Indoor and outdoor cadence ranges.* Realistic indoor cadence ranges are essential.

## Key Point

*Because of the weighted flywheel and inertia, the preferred cadence indoors will usually be 5 to 10 rpms higher.*

It is often surprising for instructors, when counting cadence indoors, to discover how easy it is to maintain a 90 rpm pedal turnover, even with appropriate resistance. Inertia, as it is related to the flywheel, is not a factor when riding outdoors. Since less-conditioned participants often prefer even higher turnovers on indoor stationary cycles, they frequently "chase the flywheel," with little or no resistance added. The only way to reduce the indoor "inertia factor" is with resistance and sound education. Once this factor is better understood, coaches can negate most of the inertia factor when riding indoors. Not all, but most momentum can be controlled by increasing the level of resistance. Preferred cadence should be established after applying enough resistance. Proper resistance optimizes conditioning.

# Coaching Riding Positions and Technique

On a properly fitted bike, cyclists know the value of staying seated. Why then, are indoor cyclists often in such a hurry to get out of the saddle? Most cyclists are more efficient when seated and climbing versus standing and climbing. It "costs" about 10 percent more energy to stand (in addition to a 5- to 10-percent increase in heart rate), when compared to staying grounded in the saddle. Because body weight is supported when seated, less energy is wasted. On a climb or during a ride, cyclists will be seated 95 percent, or more, of the time. While climbing and getting out of the saddle can be fun, effective or restorative, coaches should encourage riders to embrace the seated position (Chapter 7, *RydeTechnique*).

# Coaching Commands and Cueing at a Personal Level

Unless instructors are aware that individuals are capable of and excited about receiving coaching and implementing what they hear, most cues in the classroom are usually directed toward the class in the form of statements or questions. For example, "Lance, be sure to drive those knees forward; no side-to-side movement." That statement corrects Lance's technique error at a personal level and serves as a general technique reminder to everyone on the ride. It also allows the coach, in a variety of ways, to connect with each rider at least once during class.

Coaches who do not think that their personally directed critique/encouragement will be well-received by their riders can direct their comments to the peloton (group) and hopefully hit the intended target. For example, "Be sure to keep your knees aligned in the corridor; let's limit the side-to-side knee movement; take a look down and let's eliminate any side-to-side knee movement—and don't try this outside!"

As bits and pieces of information are added, and cueing becomes strung out, the process moves toward being ineffective, since information overload is not effective. In fact, many experienced coaches believe that early in their careers they "over-coached" their students.

**Key Point**

> *Confident coaches, who know their sport, carefully craft their cueing to be precise in the moment and specific to circumstance.*

If instructors spit out the same phrases, directed toward no one in general, no one will hear them. In fact, direct, accurate coaching closely adheres to "less is better." Superb coaching and cueing happens when instructors react to what they see. In other words, they have to be observant, focused and sensitive to how their team is riding. Effective coaching and motivational cueing can include comments that correct or acknowledge correct riding form, or both.

# 4-Com Model

RealRyder communicates using a 4-Com model—"com" being shorthand for communication. By utilizing a series of commands, questions and comments it is easy to connect with each rider, every class.

### 4-Com—four ways to effectively communicate to your classes:

1. *Direct commands to the <u>group</u> with a focused and specific message related to motivation or technique.*

   Less verbiage is better! For example:

   - "Let's do a standing posture check; just off the saddle, your weight is loaded over the pedals and off the bars."
   - "Nice…everyone is riding quiet out there, which tells me that you've got a smooth, even pedal stroke going; you're balanced over your bottom bracket, and you're light on your bars."
   - "Drill time. Let's break form on this climb for 10 seconds. This is the only time you'll ever hear me to tell you to mash and pull. Oh, doesn't that feel good, because it's easier? It's so ugly and slow. Where did our form go? Okay, time to clean up. Let's move our weight back over the saddle, off the bars, and create smooth circles again. Thirty perfect seconds, and we're over the top; stay below your threshold."

2. *Direct commands to <u>individual riders</u>—when appropriate.*

   What is good for one individual is good for all to hear. For example:

   - "Susan, unbelievable effort; good body position and smooth pedal stroke."
   - "Johnny—nice—spinning smooth circles; be sure to keep those shoulders down."
   - "Candice (aka Hammer), eyes are up—good; light smooth stroke; your shoulders are level … sweet—you're riding quiet, clean and powerfully."
   - "Bill, can you pick up a gear and keep form?"

3. *Questions that are directed toward the <u>group</u> with coaching/instructional intent.*

   For example:

   - "Should we mash?"

- "What would you do if the rider who out-sprinted you the last race has sucked onto your back wheel, and you have 500 meters until you cross the finish line?"
- "The chase group is reeling you in. What are you going to do about that?"
- "Can you keep the bike quiet and pedal stroke smooth? Okay, let's get ready to attack for 30 seconds standing."
- "Can you pick up a gear and maintain cadence?"

4. *Comments that are directed via a command, correction, question or encouraging motivational comment to each rider during every class.*

4-Com provides a structure to communicate that enables coaches to connect with all riders at a variety of levels. Instructors who use 4-Com care enough to engage with each participant on every ride. Coaches should also establish eye contact and communicate by name with each rider. Create nicknames for every team member to personalize the experience.

For example:

- "John (aka Lactate), you're dripping in a lactic acid shower. Great work!"
- "Leg Strong, you ready? It's time to stand if you're tackling this grade out of your saddle; okay, seated or standing on my cue; 15 seconds standing or seated and raising your heart rate 10 plus beats on this uncategorized climb; okay to mash and move your bike side to side … this is so steep smooth strokes are impossible. Okay, here we go gang … optional seated or standing. Let's hit it. Lead out Leg Strong. Everyone can raise their heart rate 10 beats … seated or standing. Leg Strong is taking the lactic acid bath."
- "Domestique, are you ready to pull this peloton? Domey, you're on for 30 seconds at an RPE of 7-8. Everyone else, you're sucking on his back wheel at an RPE of 4-5. Everyone, get ready for your turn to pull. Lead out Domey!"
- "Suzie … are you digging deep today? Where are you today? What will you ask of yourself on this splendid day? What will you give?" Big smile and Suzie's reply back, "I'm giving it all today, giving it all!"
- "Peloton, Whachugot?" Answer: "Always more than you!"

# Colorful Cycling Language

Injecting colorful cycling language into the rides can create a rich environment in which riders can train hard, easy, climb, learn about cycling lore, and most importantly—have fun. Appendix A, *Incorporating Authentic Cycling Language* and Chapter 14, *Creating a Ryde*, provide information on how to infuse this language into indoor rides. Instructors and riders will have fun learning the jargon that experienced cyclists use all the time.

# Encourage Association and Focus

Riding competitively is all about a mind/body connection. In that regard, RealRyder's "teach-it-real" frame of reference might be very different, compared to other fitness-centered approaches. Riders who disassociate on the road will become "road-kill" before too long. Furthermore, they will lose their training edge. A primary goal is for participants to feel the ride. Riders will thank their coaches later and will appreciate the fact that they were allowed to challenge themselves. Riders are encouraged to dig deep and feel alive for the first time, well—in maybe a long time. An important objective for coaches is to design and implement a cycling workout that is personal, challenging and level appropriate to the individual.

**Key Point**

*RealRyder participants are* always *encouraged to be "here, present and conscious."*

RealRyder coaches do *not* encourage dissociation. While dissociation might happen, it is not a desired occurrence. All too often, many members of society tend to check out with television, drugs, other addictive diversions, and far too many other unhealthy distractions. People who do not feel are not living fully. The fun and rewards of being focused and enjoying the RealRyder experience will far outweigh any potential impulse to be distracted by irrelevant activities and "going through the motions."

Coaches engage and inspire each individual to get in touch with who they are and what they feel. What a novel concept. Coaches should help their team to see the road, feel the road, embrace the sweat trickling *up* their arms, feel the pain, feel the gain, feel the accomplishment, feel the joy, feel the wind and embrace the challenge. What an experience—the thorough joy of conquering challenge and RydingReal.

The role of instructors is to set the stage—goal, duration, and intensity for each section of the ride (hills, standing, seated, breaking away, passing riders) and motivate the peloton (group) by connecting to each rider.

# 14

# Creating a Ryde:
# Planning Your Class Workouts

Many of our RealRyder cycling coaches really never wanted to come to an indoor cycling class. On the other hand, they knew that riding indoors offered certain advantages. However, they dreaded the idea of riding on a fixed stationary bike that does not move side-to-side, like a real bike. The RealRyder bike removed this objection, yet something was still missing.

The second element—and the other fundamental key to the riding philosophy and class design at RealRyder—is that almost everyone at RealRyder does not want to go to a *class.* They just wanted to *ryde.* Understandably, no one preferred a class over the real thing. The RealRyder Indoor Cycling program and bike transforms a *class* into a RealRyde.

**Key Point**

*At RealRyder, it's all about the ryde. No one has our ryde!*

The RealRyder Indoor Cycling program is designed to make planning intelligent and creative workouts easy. RealRyder brings outdoor riding information and outdoor riding indoors, yet builds on the history of indoor cycling.

## Creating a Ryde

Having a clear-cut class design methodology affects the ride experience and a coach's ability to create unlimited class rides that are unique, new and different. The methodology must be time efficient and replicable. That is why the RealRyder Indoor Cycling program can help every instructor achieve "star" status.

In order to enable instructors to diversify their teaching approach and move it beyond simply teaching proper pedaling form or cueing drills, RealRyder has developed a ryde planning system that moves teachers beyond simply instructing—to actually coaching. *Creating a Ryde* also addresses the motivational aspects of riding and helps instructors build relationships with their riders.

Standout teachers and coaches chart and plan every workout. Skilled coaches know the exact journey on which they are taking their athletes. This process is far from random. Developing this culture creates mutual respect—and in turn—athletes elevate their performance and commitment to another level. Everyone has skin in the game; everyone is invested.

Knowing the technical aspects of riding and speaking the vibrant lingo of cycling are helpful if the goals include teaching a safe, effective, diverse and results-oriented class. On the other hand, the *structure* of the class is what keeps an instructor's students coming back for more.

## Key Point

*Coaching success is defined by each and every workout. We are only as good as our last ryde!*

Our RydingPhilosophy is based on this foundation: "No one is left behind." Instructors typically have mixed ability levels that ranges from first-time indoor riders, novice riders, de-conditioned riders, fit riders who have no riding experience, to pro-cyclists. Nonetheless, all participants "ride shoulder-to-shoulder." The success of instructors and a program is often determined by how diverse of a market can be attracted, while still individualizing results and training.

## Key Point

*When personal relationships are developed, riders experience an incredible workout that manifests itself into a passion for cycling that cultivates lifelong commitment.*

World-class teaching does not happen by accident. Top-flight coaches are able to manipulate attitude, instruction, specific goals, communication/cueing and motivational strategies to get the most out of their athletes. Why should it be any different with indoor-cycling? Ongoing evaluation, shrewd manipulation and planned variety should be a part of every workout that fits into a periodized cycling program.

# General Class Design

General class design for a RydePlan should address the following:

## RydePlan

- *Bike fit and rider orientation:* Conduct a proper bike set-up for all riders; orient first-time riders to the RealRyder cycle motion.
- *Set the goal/mood of the ride:* Ascertain big-picture intensity (allocation to warm-up, drills, easy, moderate, challenging, hard) and terrain (RydeProfile).
- *Set the time:* Determine the duration of the ride; identify specific ride segments (hills, flats, standing climbs) and how long each will last.
- *Draw the RydeProfile:* Literally, draw the ups and downs of the ride, as well as horizontal elements of leaning, steering and turning.
- *Communicate the immediate focus/riding requirements:* Preview the RydeProfile.
- *Monitor the level of effort:* Explain how intensity will be monitored using rating of perceived exertion (RPE) and heart rate (HR).
- *Monitor cadence/RPM:* Explain how cadence will be monitored.
- *Cue and motivate:* RydeReal and create a positive riding experience by connecting at a personal level with each rider.
- *Focus on the entire ride:* Incorporate a philosophy that reflects the belief "How individuals start their ride is as important as how they finish."
- *Engage in long-term class planning:* Understand how classes can be periodized to meet rider needs in terms of a balanced workout approach (Chapter 17, *Periodization: Long-Term Class Planning*).

## Basic 5

Once a class has been planned using the Basic 5 elements of variation the personality and style of the coach can shine through. In terms of class planning, this is where "the rubber meets the road."

### Key Point

*Every class is focused on achieving specific, purposeful objectives.*

*Micro level coaching.* Micro level coaching involves designing a RydeProfile using the *Basic 5* (Table 14-1) and *RydeProfile Class Planning Template* (Figure 14-2) to write down and organize the workout.

*Elements of variation.* The Basic 5 elements of variation are the nuts and bolts of creative and effective ride design. Results and goal attainment (ride outcome) can endlessly be manipulated by using the five *elements of variation* to strategically plan for and accomplish the desired training result.

| Basic 5 | | | | |
|---|---|---|---|---|
| 1.<br>-Body Position<br>-Hand Placement<br>-Form | 2.<br>Load | 3.<br>Cadence | 4.<br>Bike Motion | 5.<br>RydeProfile |

Table 14-1. Basic 5 elements of variation in class planning

*CRI (cadence, resistance, intensity).* A combination of cadence and resistance/gear equate to intensity (watts or power output). How they are used will frame the quality and effectiveness of the ride, closely followed by the basic elements of variation.

Cadence + Resistance (gear) = Intensity (heart rate response, RPE, $VO_2$, watts, calories utilized)

**Key Point**

*CRI dictates the pain, the whining, the joy, the easy or hard aspects of riding, and the overall sense of achievement the rider experiences.*

# RydeProfile and Class Planning

It is important to literally visualize and sketch the RydeProfile (Figure 14-1) you are asking your participants to ride.

*Charting workouts.* All workouts should be charted—meaning preplanned and written down. RydeProfile workout records can be use to plan future workouts. Charting (see Figure 14-2, RydeProfile Class Planning Template) helps keep coach and athlete/rider accountable. Experience also shows that RealRyder participants love to repeat rides to test their mettle and measure improvement.

# Class Format

Creating a RydeProfile should largely focus on simulating rydes that incorporate the Basic 5 elements of variation.

*Simulating rides.* Using real scenarios allows you to use the race strategies and course details (e.g., elevation gain, down hills, flats, categories of climbs, type of terrain, location, etc.) that will be revealed and become part of the ride. Instructors can create an endless number of "simulated rides." At RealRyder, this strategic approach represents our favorite way of designing classes.

*Sample outdoor simulation scenario.* A favorite ride of many cyclists is the "Rock Creek Pie Ride." To get to the pie, individuals have to climb to a little restaurant at 9,373 feet of elevation. Riders from Mammoth Lakes, California make the 50-plus mile ride so they can be treated to a piece of Dutch apple, strawberry, blueberry, rhubarb or any number of other pies upon arrival. Riders have the option of continuing to Mosquito Flat, which is about a mile past the pie restaurant and adds another 1,000 feet of climbing onto an already long 12-mile climb up to Rock Creek Resort. Mosquito Flat is the highest trailhead in the Sierra Nevada, at an elevation of 10,300 ft. That extra mile at 8- to 10-percent grade, gaining 1,000 feet of elevation, at altitude, is brutal. In addition, riders are distracted by wanting the pie so badly at that point (really, they just want the rest), insult is added to injury because they must ride past the pie to get to the "flats." All is not lost, however. After that final climb and returning for their well-earned pie, an exhilarating descent that averages 40 to 50 mph awaits—assuming the rider stays off the brakes.

An example of a simulated ride on a RealRyder cycle can be illustrated by using the "Rock Creek Ride" profile from Mammoth (50 plus miles) or from the base of the climb into Rock Creek Canyon (12 miles of up!). The ride can be profiled with or without the

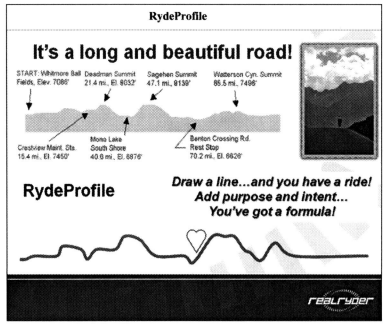

Figure 14-1. RydeProfile

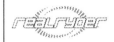

| RydeProfile Class Planning Template | | |
|---|---|---|
| **Ryde Intensity/Terrain Preview** | **Terrain Profile (draw)** | **Ryde Name/Duration** |
| | | |

| **Ryde Segment** | **Position, Terrain, Cadence** | **Intensity/ Zone** | **Coaching the Segment (key points)** | **Total Time/ Song(s)** | **Coach Notes** |
|---|---|---|---|---|---|
| I. | | | | | |
| II. | | | | | |
| III. | | | | | |
| IV. | | | | | |
| V. | | | | | |
| VI. | | | | | |
| VII. | | | | | |
| VIII. | | | | | |
| IX. | | | | | |
| X. | | | | | |
| XI. | | | | | |
| XII. | | | | | |
| XIII. | | | | | |
| XIV. | | | | | |
| XV. | | | | | |

Figure 14-2. RydeProfile class planning template

"narrows" section, and with or without the Mosquito Flat section. Instructors can also provide participants with no option and simply state— "We're riding Rock Creek with the 'narrows' and Mosquito Flat sections from the bottom of the canyon." Such a directive could be met with enthusiastic groans and unadulterated complaints from the entire class, as they embark on the 12-mile climb. Fortunately, pie *will* be provided at the end of the class. That is "real" and would only be fair!

The entire RydeProfile is patterned after what a "RealRyde" throws at participants in terms of terrain, which dictates cadence and resistance/gear. A simulated ride brings the lore and flavor of outdoor cycling to the indoor ride. During the simulated ride, instructors may even interject conversation about gear ratios and compact chain rings (e.g., by stating that "Bet you wish you had that "compact ring set-up" going through the narrows, don't you?"). The "narrows" is a difficult 8- to 12-percent grade early in the climb; it is usually hot, windless and suffocating.

Simulated rides generate interest about outdoor cycling and foster an atmosphere of accomplishment and fun. Furthermore, the experience for many participants gets better when they get a second chance to show their mettle on the same ride. Which would most riders prefer—in and out of the saddle 64 times for no apparent reason, or a ride for pie?

## RydeProfile and Class Planning Template

Figure 14-2 illustrates a proven charting tool that can accommodate all ride variables, including song selection. Open writing spaces are provided for instructor notes and comments. Taking advantage of this template is simple and can help instructors map out and preview each ride—from intensity, to cadence, to resistance/gear, body position, music and coaching cues.

*RydeProfile maps.* Researching various rides, tours and races provide instructors with an infinite number of ideas for workouts. Profiles and course maps can be used to stir up excitement and anticipation. Instructors, studios and clubs should use the buzz to market their classes. The RydeProfile process can also help keep coaches fresh. Instructors love charting and planning classes using the RydeProfile because it is quick and easy.

## Climbing Modules and Drills

It is critical to be a master at climbing. All factors being equal, riders separate on hills (and you "burn" a lot of calories). Either you have it, or you do not. This point is reinforced by the famous "look" that Lance Armstrong gave Jan Ullrich on the Alpe d'Huez at the 2001 Tour de France. Armstrong looked into Ullrich's eyes and seemed to say, "Are you coming with me or not?" The unspoken answer was a glazed and desperate look. At that moment, hill climbing separated two of the best riders in the world. Hill climbing not only "burns" a lot of calories, enhances a rider's fitness level, improves muscular strength and endurance, and builds confidence—it also represents an important skill in the sport of cycling. Being good at hill climbing is fun and gratifying.

*Climbing drills primer.* Outdoor climbing requires a slightly different body position. During seated climbs, riders should sit up straighter, with a hand position that is higher on the bars (top of bars). The higher position makes it easier to breathe and puts less stress on the rider's lower back. When climbing seated outdoors, aerodynamics is not usually important. In a standing climb position, riders are also more upright, with weight centered over the pedals and bottom bracket—hands in the "sides" position. With practice and improved technique, climbing gets easier each time participants attack a hill (Refer to Chapter 7, *RydeTechnique*).

*Rolling hill accelerations.* This drill is designed to improve power and recovery ability on rolling hills—about one to two minutes long. The series of accelerations are employed in a continuous, successive fashion, much like a steady surf break, one wave after another, up to 12 repeats for advanced riders. The drill involves having the participants ride most of the "roller" at a steady, sustainable pace. During the last 30 to 60 seconds, near the top of each hill, stand and accelerate for about 10 to 15 seconds past the top. Focus on increasing cadence to create acceleration. Recover with three to five minutes of easy riding.

The same drill can be done *seated.* Focus again, is on increasing cadence to create initial acceleration. Add gears/resistance, as needed, to increase power output.

*Overs and unders.* This drill focuses on maintaining a sustainable ride and recovery pace, but also incorporates high-intensity effort to develop power at lactate threshold heart rate (LTHR). Set the stage by telling the riders they will be doing a six-minute climb—starting at a steady and sustainable pace (below threshold but working hard) for two minutes, and then accelerating ("overs") for one minute to maximal *sustainable* pace. This effort is followed by a return to "unders" intensity for another two minutes, before accelerating again to "overs" intensity for the final minute. Do three six-minute sets/intervals with five minutes of easy recovery riding between each six-minute set. Sets can be performed using seated and standing positions. Because intensity is relative, any rider can take part in these drills.

Chapter 15, *Ryding Skills and Drills,* provides additional options.

# Colorful Cycling Language

Injecting colorful cycling language into rides can add a special dimension to the ride. Appendix A, *Incorporating Authentic Cycling Language,* and Chapter 13, *Coaching a Ryde,* provide additional information on how instructors can infuse riding language into indoor rides.

# 15

# Ryding Skills and Drills

Style and performance go hand-in-hand when riding a bike. Whether riders are sprinting, seated, out of the saddle to crest a hill, or climbing a sustained uphill effort—rhythm and finesse are the watch words, even when working hard. Good athletes make something that is relatively hard look easy. Technique drills focus on economy of movement and efficiency, as measured by how well the rider uses oxygen. An improvement in cycling skills and cardiovascular physiology equate to improved riding, pure enjoyment and better results. As skill and fitness levels increase, a greater sense of accomplishment is felt because the rider is "good"—can go longer, harder and utilize more calories. Being "good" can be stripped down to improved form, technique and fitness.

*Souplesse* occurs when the rider embraces the relationship between self and bike, as the rider and the bike respond to the natural production of forces created during each phase of the pedal stroke. This intermingling of personal style and performance helps to maximize the rider's level of riding efficiency, as the cyclist becomes ever more proficient at muscle activation and coordination on the bike.

## RydeTechnique Drills

Technique drills improve riding economy. Drills also have a neurological component, which is related to the specificity of riding. In other words, if riders are going to improve, get better, become more efficient from a skill/neuro-perspective—and utilize oxygen more efficiently—they must ride like they are going to ride. Realistic pedaling cadence, proper body position and appropriate gear/resistance are key elements.

Pedaling mechanics (Chapter 9, *Science of Cycling*) is the essence of cycling economy. The scientific aspect of pedaling economically is neural and skill based; it is not necessary to work on pedaling economy using heavy loads or pushing lactate threshold. On the other hand, some drills replicate a heavy gear/resistance or steep climb, because if riders are going to hammer out of the saddle, they must do so correctly and maintain efficiency. These drills are employed only after proper technique has been established using lighter loads. Pedaling drills require the rider to "be here, present and conscious." Riders must focus—really concentrate—on smoothness as it relates to a linked and controlled pedal stroke.

# Ryding Skills and Drills

Establishing a powerful and efficient pedal stroke requires perfect practice and repetition.

## Independent Leg Training, Single Leg Dominance, or Unweighting

The title of this section reflects the objective. Pressuring, unweighting or single-leg dominance training represent skills that are important to master when establishing pedaling economy.

*The drill set primer.* Most cyclists have detached one foot from the pedal while performing single leg drills on an indoor bike with a fixed gear; the practice should be discouraged. The risks outweigh benefit on an indoor bike. Any neurological training effect—specificity as it relates to timing and economy—is lost because of the "flywheel effect." Riders must add resistance to "feel the road," which requires them to pull the pedal up—especially when using one leg. Riders get minimal neurological specificity (muscle timing/firing) because of the flywheel momentum. As a result, the recovery phase must be "muscled" with one leg and active knee flexion. This action contradicts efficient pedaling and reinforces *incorrect* muscle activation during the pedal revolution (Chapter 9, *Science of Cycling*).

The danger of the attached foot coming loose—and either that foot or the other foot getting clubbed by a pedal—is quite real. If the rider tucks the unattached leg into the bottom bracket area, riding form is compromised. Keep both feet attached during one-leg dominance drills. This approach, coupled with focused concentration, represents "independent" leg training.

The goal of single leg training is to have each rider make a brain/muscle connection. Single leg training is not focused on pedaling fast or working hard. Riders try to improve pedaling economy by having one leg dominate, without piggybacking on what the other leg is doing. Doing so rids the stroke of any weak links. With the feet clipped into the pedals, the rider identifies differences between what each leg is doing independently/differently of the other.

## Independent Leg Drills

*Note:* Both legs are clipped in or otherwise attached to the pedals for all drills.

- *Single-leg pressure drill.* Riders accelerate the power phase leg, from 2 to 4 o'clock. They feel bottom dead center and create a pulling back action. During the recovery phase, the leg is unweighted and "light" on the pedal. Still pulling up and back—but NOT pulling the *pedal* up—the goal is to stay ahead of pedal velocity. Once the stroke is understood, alternately focus on the "power push" over the top and then switch the focus to "unweighting" the pedal during the recovery phase.
- *Single leg pressure drill variation.* Employ the same basic fundamentals of the previous drill; riders choose very specific parts of the pedal stroke on which to focus. For example, 12 versus 6, 3 versus 9, and so on.
- *Unilateral (dead-leg) stroke drill.* One leg is going along for the ride, and though attached to the pedal, does not contribute to the pedal stroke. Riders should focus on the entire pedal revolution using one leg dominance. Switch legs.
- *Simultaneous pressure drill.* Riders choose different parts of the pedal stroke on which to focus—for example, 12 and 6, 3 and 9. Focus on how the power and recovery leg work when the legs are positioned in opposition to one another. Switch leg emphasis with regard to power and recovery phases.

Single leg dominance drills have considerable impact with regard to improving pedaling mechanics and power output. These drills can play an essential role in helping to create physical (strength) and neural (coordination) equality between the legs.

## Clock Drills

Riders visualize pedal stroke as the face of a clock. The rider associates the face of the clock with different parts of the pedal stroke that must be linked to create a smooth pedal stroke. Using too little load is ineffective and can cause an up-and-down (i.e., piston) motion, which is in contrast to a correct circular motion.

The pedal stroke should be broken down into five phases and emphasize a front-to-back motion:

- 10 o'clock to 2 o'clock: Drive forward and over the top.
- 2 o'clock to 4 o'clock: The key part of the power phase; the highest force that is transferred to the pedal occurs at the 3 o'clock position.
- 12 o'clock to 6 o'clock: The 180-degree power phase.
- 6 o'clock to 9 o'clock: The bottom or bottom dead center (6 o'clock) and where "unloading of the pedal" begins to occur.
- 6 o'clock to 12 o'clock: The 180-degree recovery phase.

Any aspect of the clock's face/pedal stroke can be emphasized. For example, 10-2 aligns with knee extensor (quadriceps) muscle activity; 12-5 with hip extensor (gluteus maximus and hamstrings) activity; 4-9 knee flexor (hamstrings and gastrocnemius) activity; and 7-12 hip flexor (rectus femoris, iliacus, psoas) activity, which occurs during the recovery or unweighting phase. As focus shifts from right to left leg—key in on any differences/weaknesses that exist between the legs. Riders should also drive the knees forward on each leg and not let either knee drive inside/outside into an "egg beater" motion. Driving one or both knees in an inside/out pattern creates orthopedic stress on the knee joint and is inefficient in terms of force application.

## Pulling-Back Drill

Emphasize the bottom of the pedal stroke using a pulling back motion (e.g., somewhat similar to pushing back off the ground while riding a skateboard). Riders should focus on the pedal stroke at bottom dead center to train the hamstrings (neuro-component) to fire a fraction of a second faster at the bottom of the stroke—so that they do not "waste time" pushing heavily *down,* rather than driving the pedal *back and around.* Working this drill can help eliminate bouncing in the saddle that occurs either because of too much down force when pedaling at fast cadences, or as a result of riders who pedal too fast to control pedal speed.

## Draw a Circle (Link It Up Drill)

Drawing circles teaches correct force application to the pedal—not too heavy, not too light and not at all. The primary objective of the drill is to connect the dots in a way that creates a smooth pedal stroke synergy. The line thickness (amount of pressure on the pedal) being drawn should remain consistent. If riders push too heavily on the down stroke power phase, the line thickens. If they pull up too aggressively during the up stroke recovery phase, the line thickens. If they get too lazy over the top and from 2 to 4 o'clock, the line gets thinner here or disappears. Finally, if a bobble or hitch occurs either at the top or bottom of the stroke, a jag occurs in the circle that needs to be eliminated. Riders are sometimes asked to envision that they have a pen inserted into the outside of the pedal axle and that the pen is drawing a circle during the pedal revolution on poster board. Ask, "What kind of circle is being etched?

## Train—aka "Loco-Mo" Drill

It is not uncommon for instructors to preach, "Drive the legs like an old locomotive train." The engine car had a "drive train"—the horizontal bars attached to the wheels of the train. When riders drive their legs like an old locomotive (Loco-Mo), it keeps the knees driving toward the middle to inside of the bars, rather than out. Simultaneously, this action serves as a reminder that the wheels of a train go 'round and round'—never changing their pattern.

## Climbing Drills

With practice every cyclist can climb like a pro. Chapter 14, *Creating a Ryde,* provides several excellent climbing workouts.

## Cadence Drills

Anything that connects to cadence affects riding form. Cadence drills focus on leg speed development, which is highly trainable. Cadence should be "trained" weekly.

*Bounce threshold drill.* Bouncing in the saddle should be avoided for any number of reasons, including pedal stroke is incorrect. When bouncing in the saddle happens, riders need to slow down by adding load and control pedal speed. The drill is not designed to encourage bouncing in the saddle, but rather, to eliminate it. Riders should start at a preferred cadence (note for reference) or about 80 rpm, at an RPE of 4-6. Subsequently, pedal cadence should be increased by about 5 rpm every 30 to 60 seconds and RPE maintained. A rider often bounces because the hamstrings are not firing fast enough to drive the pedal backwards, which causes the rider to dominate the power phase of the pedal stroke with a hard finishing/mashing action (up and down) at the bottom (6 o'clock) of the pedal stroke. When the power phase foot hits the bottom of the stroke the hips are pushed up off the seat. Neural factors (hamstrings firing too slowly), pedaling too fast and a lack of adequate resistance are all major contributors to "bouncing in the saddle."

*Cadence pyramiding drills.* A number of drills use a pyramiding concept. In this instance, cadence and pedal stroke are the focus. One day focus on an rpm range from 60 to 110, depending on the participant's "bounce threshold." Generally, 3 to 5 rpm increments every three minutes works well. Note that three minutes is usually enough time for the heart rate and RPE, as it relates to effort, to reach a steady state or adjust to the increased workload. This drill is usually capped at 120 rpm. Very few riders can exceed this cadence, maintain pedal control and keep from bouncing in the seat. Focus on a narrow cadence range—within 60 to 110—to fine tune the rider's sense of cadence and form at different rpm.

*Cadence accelerations or spin-ups.* Accelerations focus on how riders reach a desired rpm. For example, riders might start at 80 rpm and gradually increase cadence to 100 rpm in 60 seconds. Using the same example, riders could start in a seated position at 80 rpm and accelerate to 100 rpm in a standing position within a few seconds—being sure to encourage adequate resistance when transitioning out of the saddle. In either example, riders could hold the highest level of rpm for a set number of seconds, but keep it realistic. The drill is not designed to be a torture or survival exercise. Riders can remain seated or stand, depending on the goal.

**Key Point**

*The various combinations of cadence, resistance/gears and body position intertwine—and represent all that IS cycling.*

# 16

# Mobility Training for the Cyclist

Flexibility is an important, yet often neglected component of cycling. Without adequate flexibility—smooth and easy performance of everyday and recreational activities would be impossible. Muscles should be stretched after a warm-up and preferably at the end of a workout. Static stretching post workout is the preferred method of flexibility training for most people. Injury risk is low and static stretching requires relatively little time or assistance. A dynamic mobility warm-up pre cycling is not required, but remains an option.

The muscle groups used during a ride should be targeted in the post cool-down stretching segment. Focus stretching on the calves, hamstrings, quadriceps, hip flexors, gluteals, back, chest, triceps and neck. Each stretch should be held at a point of tightness—comfortably uncomfortable without pain—for 15 to 30 seconds.

*Cycling specific flexibility.* Cycling is a lower body dominant activity, but flexibility in the major muscles of the body must be addressed. Proper body positioning while riding is designed to absorb forces, streamline mechanics and help to create an effective pedal stroke. Rounded shoulder and low back positioning can be addressed by targeted stretching and using an upright position. Another downside to a static cycling position is that it does not allow for rotary action of the spine. A comprehensive stretching program will not only stretch the muscles and joints in flexed and extended positions, but also include rotary movements.

*Bottom line application.* It is essential that cyclists engage in a complete stretching program post ride that counters "stress positions" on the bike. Target the muscles of the hips and knees that are continually used in a constrained range-of-motion because of the pedal stroke—which restricts greater or less movement. When cycling, the knee, as is true for the hip, is never fully extended or flexed. Accordingly, stretches that counter restricted movement or sustained position are included in the following section.

# Mobility Training

Recommended stretching exercises can be performed on or off the bike.

## Stretches on the RealRyder Bike

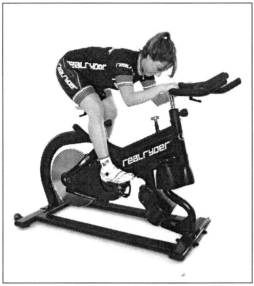

Figure 16-1. Aerodynamic descent position (low back and hip extensors)

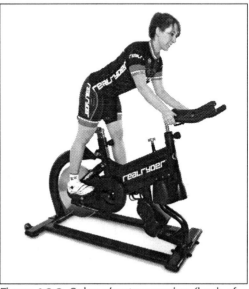

Figure 16-2. Soleus/gastrocnemius (back of the lower leg)

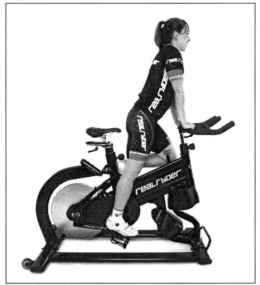

Figure 16-3. Standing hip flexor (front of the hip)

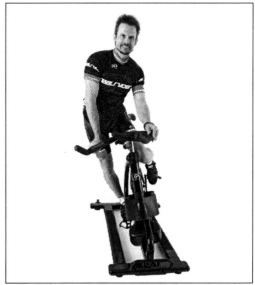

Figure 16-4. Iliotibial band (outside of the hips)

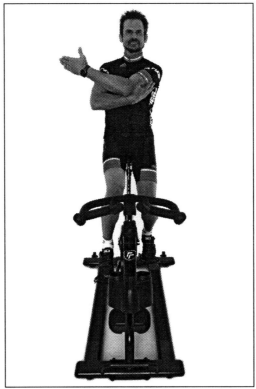

Figure 16-5. Seated back of the triceps/ shoulder (back of the shoulder)

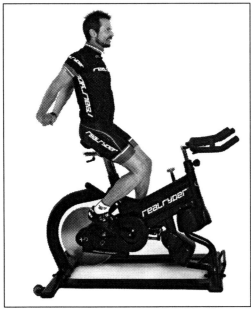

Figure 16-6. Seated anterior deltoids (front of the shoulder)

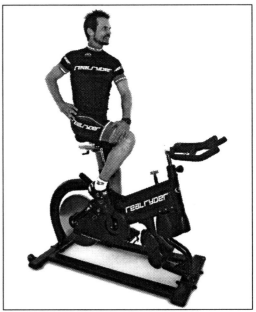

Figure 16-7. Rotary torso

## Stretches off the RealRyder Bike

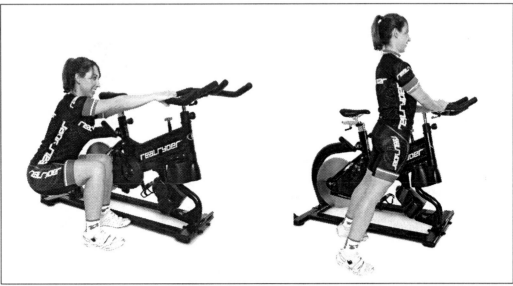

Figure 16-8. Side-of-bike standing series (*Note:* Each of the hip stretches that are included in the standing series can also be performed independently.)

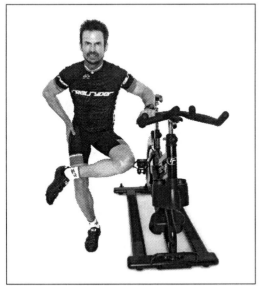

Figure 16-9. Hip adductors/internal rotators and hip extensors

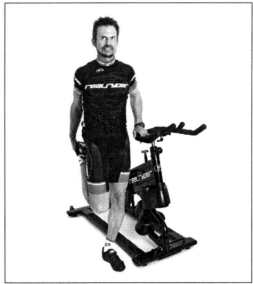

Figure 16-10. Quadriceps/hip flexors

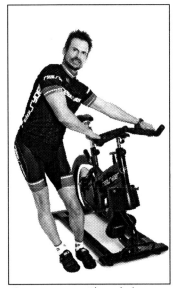

Figure 16-11. Gluteals/
IT-band

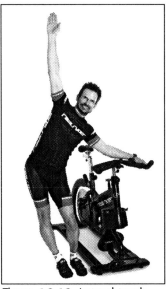

Figure 16-12. Lateral trunk

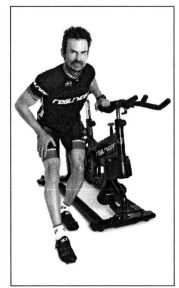

Figure 16-13. Hamstrings

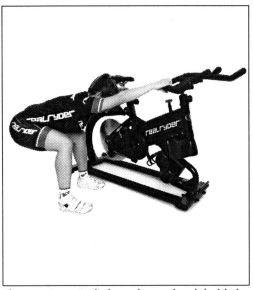

Figure 16-14. Latissimus/posterior deltoids/
triceps

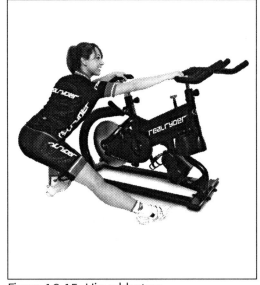

Figure 16-15. Hip adductors

# 17

# Periodization— Long-Term Class Planning

Periodization can be defined as varying workout intensity over specific time periods. Another way to look at periodizing an indoor cycling schedule is to focus on "long-term class planning."

## Key Point

*Periodization moves beyond planning a single ride and recognizes the training needs of an individual rider as it relates to intensity changes and overall ride variety.*

While it is important to acknowledge periodization—rather than attempt the impossible and attempt to create a class schedule that meets everyone's individual training needs—the key is to know what class participants are doing with regard to other workouts. Riders should be encouraged to carefully choose the classes that will enable them to effectively plan and balance their overall workout approach. It is the responsibility of participants to craft a sensible and balanced approach to their workouts. The role of the coach is to guide them.

*Long-term class planning.* For coaches and instructors, the big picture (e.g., macro-level of planning cycling rides and class schedule) looks at class needs over a longer period of time and its impact, as well as its appeal to class participants or outdoor cyclists.

No matter how well instructors plan and schedule their classes, and diversify ride content, these efforts will *not* result in perfectly matching to *all* class participant needs.

Why participants enroll in a class can range from the instructor's personality, weight loss, stress release, non-impact workout, endurance, recovery rides, interval training or preparing for an upcoming century ride—to name a few. If enough classes were offered riders could choose classes based on training goals, needs, desire or mood of the day. Some will take the same class, regardless of what is being taught, based on *who* is leading the ride. Others will attend classes at the same time, regardless of *what* is being taught, because that time is convenient. Though a perfect world does not exist, instructors should make every effort to be creative and accommodating with regard to class schedules and themes.

This "reality factor" does not equate to throwing in the towel. Instructors should still query students with regard to how they introduce variety into their long-term workout schedule. Getting a perspective of what riders are and are not doing—and understanding *why* and *when* they attend RealRyder cycling classes—can positively influence the teaching schedule.

## Key Point

*Instructors should teach their riders how to be responsible for overall workout balance.*

*What instructors can do.* Instructors have an unlimited number of options at their disposal for keeping sessions fresh and providing what the customer needs. Consider a schedule where an instructor has a class scheduled Monday, Wednesday and Friday at 6 a.m. Not surprisingly, some of the same riders will regularly attend. If that is true, careful planning will be required to keep these riders challenged and interested. One possible solution would be for the instructor to plan a month's worth of workouts (12 rides) and let the group know the plan for the next month. If a first-time attendee arrives for a class that has an intense interval workout planned, the individual can be guided accordingly.

Other class offerings may involve a more "random" type of scheduling. For example, classes might be offered at 10 a.m., 12 noon, and 6:30 p.m. Some or none of the scheduled classes may be repeated. A variety of instructors might instruct the same time slot on different days. In this instance, riders should be taught to choose which class to attend, based on what type of workout is being planned. Instructors who offer a season based schedule of class offerings can plan spring workouts that emphasize endurance and base building workouts for cyclists who are looking to "get their legs back" for the outdoor riding season.

## Key Point

*Instructors should clearly brand their classes with regard to intensity level and duration so that participants can choose the ride that matches workout needs and optimizes training efforts.*

# Periodization Primer

Balanced physical programming walks a fine line between listening to what riders want to do and incorporating those interests into a program that also addresses what *needs* to get done!

Riders are encouraged to:

*Schedule workouts.* Scheduling means commitment and commitment means success. Scheduled workouts should be honored as an important covenant. This commitment should be viewed no differently by individuals when compared to a meeting with a boss or prospective client.

*Identify the best time to work out.* This is not complex. The best time has nothing to do with a person's metabolism, circadian and biological rhythms, or the body's daily ups and downs. Individuals should choose the time to exercise when it best aligns with personality. If you hate rising early—forget scheduling early morning workouts.

**Key Point**

*The best time for individuals to work out is the time at which they will get it done!*

# Planning Workouts: Periodization Made Easy

A periodized program varies how hard, how much, how often and the types of activity in which a person engages—over specific time periods. Periodization encourages riders to introduce change and purposeful variety into their training program.

**Key Point**

*Periodization is simply defined as "planned results."*

Periodization has the potential to:

- Promote optimal response to the training stimulus or work effort.
- Decrease the potential for overuse injuries.
- Keep riders fresh and progressing toward achieving their training goal(s).
- Optimize each participant's personal efforts.
- Enhance compliance.

## Principles of Periodization

Periodization is a method to organize training. A periodized program cycles volume (minutes, distance, duration) and intensity (load, force, resistance, speed, cadence/rpm) over specific time periods. The underlying science of periodization involves achieving optimal intensity (stress) and recovery (restoration). Of these two key aspects—intensity and recovery—neither is more important than the other. Each must be given equal emphasis.

*Comparing athletes to fitness enthusiasts.* The most obvious difference between elite athletes and most fitness participants is that the need to "peak" for performance is minimal or nonexistent for the latter. For athletes, maximal performance generally coincides with important competitions. As a result, the change that fitness enthusiasts undergo from one phase of training to another will be more subtle than for high-level athletes. The training phases for "average" participants involve three basic stages—preparation or buildup, goal attainment and restoration/recovery. Active people who have already achieved their desired level of fitness may have several program goals, including engaging in a variety of activities, solidifying their current fitness levels and establishing a commitment to exercise on a regular basis.

### Key Point

*Ongoing evaluation of the needs and goals of individuals is a necessity, whether they are just starting an exercise program or have already attained a high level of fitness.*

A well-planned periodized program addresses short-, mid- and long-term needs. Such a planning process considers daily workouts (microcycles of about 7 to 10 days), an agenda that accounts for three to four weeks (six to eight weeks for highly trained athletes) of training (mesocycles), and an overall annual training scheme, or at least several months of planning (macrocycle). After every three to four weeks of progressive overload, riders should incorporate at least several workouts of active recovery into their training schedule. Active recovery (active "rest") is usually undertaken at lower intensities of effort and duration than previous exercise levels. Riders should also consider engaging in different activities (cross-train), at least part of the time, for their recovery and restoration time periods.

Once planned results have been achieved, the intensity of effort or load can be determined for the next phase. This cyclic process determines the contents and organization of the programming process.

## Periodization Model for Health and Fitness

The following five-step process can be employed to plan a periodized, goal-oriented indoor-cycling training program:

❑ Step #1: Establish the goal(s) of the program:

- Cardiovascular goals
- Muscular strength and endurance goals
- Flexibility goals
- Other goals (e.g., set a new personal record (best) in the next bike race, prepare for a century ride, or complete a bike race)

❑ Step #2: Determine how to achieve the goal(s) of the program:

- Assess time availability
- Identify types (mode) of activity (e.g., indoor cycling, weight training, yoga, etc.)
- Match training to goals
- Choose preferred activities

❑ Step #3: Identify training phases and create an exercise plan:

- *Training phases:*
  - Develop 3 to 10 day short-term planning (microcycle).
  - Develop a three to four week training plan (mesocycle).
  - Develop a yearly organizational training plan (macrocycle), or at least three to four months of mesocycles.
  - Plan a general preparation phase of three to four weeks (one mesocycle), which may be repeated several times.
- *Exercise Plan:*
  - Manipulate the frequency, intensity and duration of each activity to achieve specific results in the body's energy and physiologic systems.
  - Apply appropriate principles of frequency, intensity and duration to each fitness component in the general preparation and goal phase.
  - Achieve the intended results by adhering to proper intensity of effort (load) and planning in adequate recovery (restoration).

❑ Step #4: Plan volume and intensity (overload):

- *Vary volume and overload on a cyclic basis:*
  - Change the duration and overload every three to four weeks at a minimum, and/ or within a 3 to 10 day microcycle.
  - Plan to increase or decrease duration and intensity.

- Use lower intensities and less duration during restoration (active rest).
- Start the new mesocycle, after active recovery, at a slightly lower level of intensity than the previous cycle.

- *Allow for the restoration/recovery process:*
  - In general, do not increase progressive overload for more than three continuous weeks.
  - Follow any sustained, progressive three to four week (mesocycle) increase in overload with at least several days of active recovery at a lower level of intensity. The effort should be less intense compared to the last overload phase.
  - After active recovery start the new mesocycle at a slightly lower level of intensity than the previous cycle and build from that point.

❏ Step #5: Regularly evaluate the periodization planning process:

- Monitor results and progress of the program.
- Employ fitness assessments (optional).
- Recognize achievement of program goals.
- Observe compliance and enthusiasm toward the program.

# Stage 3

## Rolling In

# 18

# Music: Along for the Ryde!

Love it or hate it—depends on music style and preferences. Get it right, everyone loves it. Music *can* become—"choreography" of sorts. It can serve as a roadmap for the ride. Or, as we say, the *ride serves as the road map and music goes along for the ride.* This flip-flop makes music no less important, but it is a distinction. Music does *not* create the ride. Participants do not ride fast or slow, in a big or small gear, while seated or standing—because of the music.

**Key Point**

*"I only ask one thing of music; does it motivate me to ride?"*

It can be argued that outdoor riders do not get out of the saddle because of a song. They stand because the "road turns up" or they want to "gap" an opponent. The ride comes first, the music second. Instructors should develop the RydeProfile/terrain features and identify training goals. Then—look to music to enhance the energy and emotion of the ride.

**Key Point**

*Music should not dictate what an individual does on their bike. Ride goals, opponents, and terrain dictate riding response.*

Music tempo should not dictate how a hill is climbed! Rather, instructors should plan the ride first and align what they are trying to accomplish with music. All instructors should be fully aware of the power of music to encourage and motivate.

Music can create an amazing energy level. It can motivate riders to set and keep a pace they normally could not sustain. Turn work into play. No one should underestimate the impact that music can have during an indoor or outdoor ride.

**Key Point**

*When the energy of music syncs up with an emotion that drives riders, it can be very powerful, to say the least.*

*Music is intensely personal.* To individual cyclists, music can be viewed on a continuum of attitudes—from very annoying to absolutely perfect. For intensely focused riders, music is typically viewed as a distraction from the task at hand. But, this feeling can vary day to day. Obviously, preferences change based on the ride. One person's motivation can be another's dread. Riding to music rhythm for a couple of songs can also work, rather than having music drive the response for an entire ride. Riders who cycle on the beat should ride clean and smooth, driving through, not stomping on the beat.

# Music

An instructor's music preferences and style of teaching will largely determine the type of music used indoors. Some instructors believe that music is important for setting the mood of the workout, but not for keeping pace to or dictating response. Other instructors use music to establish cadence and synch the class. RealRyder recommends instructors not teach a class designed solely around beats per minute (BPM) and take into consideration the general music preferences of the group.

**Key Point**

*The focus on music should be for motivational purposes, rather than a choreographed countdown.*

*Utilizing music.* Instructors who create their own playlists will probably love every song. A particular song can send individuals "flying" or lull them into recovery mode. Music can signal a warm-up, flat terrain, pumping up a hill, slipping through valleys on a brilliant sunny day, powering up steep climbs, descending a fast downhill at breakneck speeds, cornering a sharp turn or cooling down in a soft rain after a hard ride (e.g., *Riders on the Storm*—The Doors).

*Note:* Instructors must adhere to regulations as pertains to individual and commercial use of music.

For some instructors, music is the difference between a good and great class. However, we believe an exceptional instructor and our ryde makes the difference between a good and great class. An individual does not have to be a disc-jockey to lead an amazing class. Good or outstanding music can be a part of a great ride. Instructors should not lean too heavily on music. Instead, take the class for a ryde and teach them something that will enhance the experience. An emotional experience does not have to occur every ryde. Students are not looking for another workout that is a "choreographed count down." They really "want to ryde." Students should end the class and comment, "Hey coach, *great* ryde! Thanks! Oh—*good* music, too!"

*Music type.* Instructors should consider the music preferences of their students. "Top 40" music tends to work well, as do remixes from popular songs of the past. Since remixes are often longer, it is easier to piece together longer riding sections without the distraction of a music lull. Music without lyrics offers an advantage, because the coach does not have to compete with song lyrics. Sometimes lyrics work and sometimes they do not. Different styles of music have different bpm ranges, which affects how the song might be used for cadence. Rhythm can also vary within a song from high to low energy, or remain fairly steady throughout the song. Regardless, the song must work for what the instructor is trying to accomplish during the ride. Finally, and most important, does the song make you want to ride that section?

**Key Point**

*Instructors should set the RydeProfile and goals, and then look to music for whatever it can contribute in terms of motivation and energy.*

*Music mapping.* Music mapping is for instructors "who know their music." In other words, they listen to each song in their playlist that they have selected for a particular ride and then detail (map) what happens in the song and what should occur on the ride during each noteworthy segment of the song. For example, instructors would pinpoint how long the "soft intro" lasted, what they would teach during that intro, followed by the next segment, and so on. However, instructors are not always able to achieve a perfect match between the song's basic characteristics and the riding goals of the class. As discussed previously—songs should not dictate the ride.

Frankly, it is odd that many instructors tend to teach each song as a ride in of itself, starting with a mellow beginning and finishing with a big ending. Then, "it" starts over again on the next song. That scenario is a class—rather than a ryde—and simply involves a number of individual workout segments. Such a class indicates little thinking has gone into the RydeProfile in terms of what is, and is not, being accomplished. That is not RealRyding.

It can be argued that nothing is wrong with a workout for the sake of a workout; it is better than nothing. On the other hand, considerable benefits can be derived from being more precise from a planning perspective over the course of a year (periodization). If the song fits the RydeProfile—drill(s), terrain or the competitor's response—take advantage of it. Some instructors spend too much time with music selection, teach a class—and miss the ryde!

Always working on the beat can make cycling restrictive or inappropriate for many riders, as well as eliminate some benefits and fun. Pre-set cadence—based on song bpm—can be too easy, too hard or simply not match the ride or preferred cadence. One cadence or beat does not match up to all fitness and skill capabilities, or what is natural to some cyclists. If students try to maintain a cadence that is too fast, they might lower resistance to inappropriate levels and ride with poor form. Instructors should always employ a "preferred cadence option," rather than a predetermined cadence (music rhythm).

Music has features that go well beyond musical beat, such as rhythm and the use of specific instruments. In fact, many riders cannot hear 8-count or 32-count phrasing, but they are able to get as much joy out of music whether they are on the beat or not, whether they are synced to the rhythm or not. The joy of movement and rhythm come from within. All factors considered—participants should "ryde to their own beat."

**Key Point**

*Everyone can ryde to—and benefit from—the emotion of music.*

# 19

# Ryding Comfort and Injury Prevention

New riders regularly complain of discomfort in the hands, wrists, feet, buttocks, upper back and low back. A number of these issues can be eliminated by proper bike fit, appropriate cadence, adequate resistance and correct riding form. On the other hand, cyclists sometimes simply need enough "seat time" to alleviate some "aches." General discomfort diminishes with time spent on the bike.

Riders must distinguish between discomfort and pain. The former is the body's message communicating "this is different," while the latter is the body signaling that "something is wrong." The difference between discomfort and sharp pain can be minimal in some instances, but injury/safety implications are substantial.

To prevent unnecessary discomfort or an unwarranted risk of injury on the bike, special attention must be paid to posture, riding form and bike fit. Many of the complaints that are reported involving discomfort and overuse injuries in the neck, upper shoulders, arms, wrists, low-back and feet can be traced to poor riding form, incorrect or unchanging hand position, or bad posture. Adequate hydration, functional cycle clothing and shoes, and an appropriate warm-up and cool-down are essentials. Riders must remember that a fixed-gear bike does not allow for a free-spin. The crank continues to turn unless it is controlled to a stop.

*Numbness/discomfort in the hands/wrists or feet.* Numbness occurs when blood flow to an area of the body is limited or the nerves to that area are compressed. When riders grip the handlebars too tightly or allow too much body weight to push down on the hands, circulation may be compromised. Participants should be reminded to relax the hands and place them lightly on the handlebars. The wrists should be "rolled" to a neutral position. Frequently shifting the hands from one position to another on the bars can prevent numb hands or pain. Riders should keep the upper body relaxed and elbows flexed. The slight elbow bend acts as a shock absorber and relieves pressure on the hands. Numb or sore feet may be caused by pedal straps that are too tight, feet that are jammed into the shoe cage too far, clenched toes or improperly fitting shoes. Clip-in cycling shoes are highly recommended for comfort and performance. Foot pain or numbness can also result from wearing soft-soled shoes. Specially designed cycling shoes that have stiffer soles distribute pressure evenly over the pedal, in addition to helping riders pedal more efficiently. Too much resistance/gear can also cause foot pain because more pressure is exerted where the foot connects to the pedal.

*Sore/numb buttocks.* It is common for participants who are new to cycling to complain of soreness or numbness in the buttocks area, until the buttocks becomes accustomed to the pressure applied when riding. As cyclists become more skilled at riding, they can shift slightly forward or back during seated riding and stand when they need a break from being seated. Padded bike shorts are a "must have" and a soft-seat cover can be helpful. Improper cycle clothing (wearing gym shorts) can cause saddle sores. Cycling shorts are typically made without seams and no underwear layering, which eliminates sources of chafing and pressure points. While it may seem contradictory, as ride-time increases, a narrow/harder saddle is more comfortable than a fat/cushy seat. Riders should change position on/off the seat as needed; it "feels great" to stand for a few seconds after extended bouts of seated riding. Give it time; it will get better.

*Back discomfort and neck pain.* New riders should set the handlebars above seat height. Riders with back or neck problems should begin with the handlebars as high as is necessary to ride comfortably.

Complaints of numbness in the hands or pain in the neck, arms or shoulders can indicate that the handlebars are too low. Raising them can help take stress off these areas of the body and can provide a more comfortable ride. Improper bike set-up (stretched out too far), as well as tight hamstrings and hip flexors, can cause neck pain by forcing the spine to round or arch and the neck to hyperextend.

## Comfort and Injury Prevention Based on Proper Bike Fit

This section is designed for coaches who are interested in more detail behind a high performance or custom fit. Chapters 5 and 6, *Bike Fit* and *Ryde Orientation Recipe,* offer additional information on the subject.

*Seat height.* Research on knee pain during cycling has found that the correct seat height for individuals with no knee pain allows for 25 to 30 degrees of flexion of the extended leg—when the pedal is at bottom dead center. This range of knee flexion allows adequate decompression of the knee, which helps prevent anterior knee injuries, and helps avoid the "dead spot" at the bottom of the pedal stroke. Seats that are too high can cause posterior knee pain and can create hip rock side-to-side, whereas seats that are too low or too far forward can lead to anterior knee pain.

*Bike set-up tips.* All riders are unique; participants may need to readjust seat height after initial set-up. Any changes should be done in small increments. Tables 19-1 and 19-2 highlight factors that impact proper bike fit and comfort.

| Personal factors | Solution |
|---|---|
| Length of the rider's feet | Long feet have the effect of lengthening the legs. Riders with feet that are long for their height may need to raise seat height. |
| Excessive soft tissue in the gluteal region | Cyclists with excessive soft tissue (i.e., fat or muscle) over their sit bones may need to lower the seat height. However, when the rider sits for awhile the soft tissue compresses. |
| Shoe thickness | Insoles or cycling orthotics that extend under the ball of the foot have the effect of adding length to the legs. The seat height may need to be raised. |
| Space between the crotch and the seat | Adding thickness between the rider and the seat—when wearing padded cycling shorts or using a padded seat cover—effectively shortens the legs. This outcome may require a lower seat height. But, the material can compress during the ride. |

Table 19-1. Optimal seat height considerations

| Problem | Correction |
|---|---|
| Hips rocking in seated position | The seat position may be too high. Lower the seat in small increments until hips remain level during pedaling. |
| Inadequate knee extension | The seat position is too low. Raise the seat in small increments until knee flexion range is between 10 and 40 degrees of the extended leg at bottom dead center—25 to 30 degrees may be optimal. |

Table 19-2. Seat height troubleshooting tips

*Handlebar height and fore/aft position.* Upper body position and riding comfort are closely related to handlebar height. The upper body posture adopted by a "serious" cyclist tends to be a function of comfort, performance, experience, hamstrings and trunk/torso flexibility, back related problems, and the ability to rotate the hips. For professional cyclists posture is focused on performance—not whether or not it is "good for you." New riders should start with the handlebars above seat height. As participants gain more experience and become more comfortable on the bike, they can be encouraged to lower their handlebars to seat height. However, because aerodynamic factors indoors (wind resistance) are not important, lowering the handlebar height is more relevant to riders who prefer to replicate outdoor-specific riding posture. Riders with back problems should begin with their handlebars as high as is comfortable, advice that also holds true for recreational riders.

"Arm reach" is perfected when adjusting fore/aft bar position. If the elbows are completely extended when the hands are in the "sides" position, the bars should be moved closer to the rider. If too much bend exists in the elbow (e.g., more than slight elbow flexion) the bars should be moved away from the rider. If this correction is made by sliding the *seat* forward or back, doing so will have a negative impact on proper knee/foot positioning that was set during the individual's bike fit. Be sure to slide the bars, not the seat, when dialing in "arm reach."

Complaints of numbness in the hands or pain in the neck, arms or shoulders may indicate that the handlebars are too low. Raising them can help take pressure off the hands, which is re-directed to these areas by compensatory adjustments in riding posture. In addition, reminding participants to maintain a neutral wrist position can help prevent wrist discomfort and potential overuse injury. Frequent hand position changes can minimize hand discomfort and numbness.

# Common Injury Sites and Prevention Checklist

❑ Knees

- bike fit; tibial rotation/floating pedals; resistance; body awareness

❑ Lower back region

- discomfort/strain often result of sustained trunk flexion
- change bike fit; height of bars; change body position; use anterior and posterior pelvic tilt during ride; hinge at hip, rather than flexing spine

❑ Neck

- strengthen; more upright posture, with eyes focused ahead; alignment; neutral neck position

❑ Wrists and forearms

- change position frequently; strengthen; stretch

❑ Saddle soreness

- padded bike shorts; progression/toughen the buttocks area; anatomical seats, which accommodate wider hip bones; correct seat height; frequently change position of buttocks/pubis bone on seat

❑ Stabilization/functional strength

- off-bike conditioning

❑ Postural awareness

- correct body alignment; posture checks

# Safety While Ryding

Pedal control and adequate resistance are necessary for skilled and safe riding.

*Maintaining pedal control.* Participants of varying skill and fitness levels can slip out of pedal straps or release from the pedal when clipped in—causing a loss of control. The rider must react by clearing the leg(s) and follow this action by quickly stopping the flywheel. Not allowing participants to pedal out of control and instructing them to always have adequate resistance are two safety measures that can help prevent this scenario. Each rider should receive instruction and reminders on how to control cadence and stop quickly if necessary. The RealRyder cycle is equipped with a safety stop that can be used in situations where the rider loses foot contact with a pedal(s) and needs to regain control quickly. The safety stop can be activated by firmly pushing the red resistance knob downward.

Riders should be cautioned to always work with the right amount of resistance even during flat sections, cadence drills, warm-up or cool-down. Resistance ensures that the soft tissues surrounding the knee joint are protected from momentous forces created by a fast-spinning flywheel. This protection is achieved by activating the leg musculature to control the pedal, rather than the pedal controlling the rider. Having resistance on the flywheel enables the rider to maintain control of the pedaling motion and sustain proper riding form.

# Pre-Ride Maintenance and Safety Check

Maintenance is an ongoing battle with bikes that are heavily used. Simple and quick to complete, maintenance is absolutely essential for continued high performance and safety of participants. Conducting bike checks on a regular basis is the foundation of a successful preventive maintenance program.

Maintenance checks include:

❑ Check that all adjustment knobs are fully tightened after proper set-up is established.

❑ Check that the base of the bike is level; use adjustable leveling feet.

❑ Check that the chain is lubricated and adjusted properly.

❑ Check that the emergency stop/resistance knob is adjusted properly and functions as intended.

❑ Check that the bike is operating smoothly and quietly before each ride.

❑ Regular maintenance should be performed following the recommendations in the *RealRyder Indoor Cycling Owner's Manual.*

# 20

# Ventilation, Hydration and Fueling

Riding outdoors provides a cyclist with the advantage of wind passing over the body to help dissipate sweat. But—a controlled, consistent and perfect indoor environment is possible.

Wind created naturally or by forward movement helps sweat evaporate and keep the body cool. Riders tend to sweat more indoors because of limited air circulation. Air circulation and its cooling effect indoors can be increased by strategically placing fans. Adequate ventilation can be achieved by using a central heating/cooling system and/ or opening windows to improve air flow. Temperature and humidity must be properly managed.

*Fluid intake.* To prevent dehydration and aid body temperature regulation, participants should drink fluids before, during and after class. Bring two water bottles along for the ride. Replacing fluids as they are lost keeps the body hydrated, improves performance and facilitates recovery. Staying hydrated can increase the "enjoyment factor" and decrease perceived effort level. Participants will experience a lower RPE (rating of perceived exertion) for the *same* ride, if they hydrate.

**Key Point**

*Optimal hydration is the replacement of fluid, calories and electrolytes based on individual needs.*

A properly formulated sport drink is an effective hydration beverage that can help replace fluids *and* electrolytes (including sodium and potassium) lost in sweat by sustaining the physiological drive to drink and by helping maintain fluid homeostasis. For any class ride that pushes an hour, participants should consider consuming an electrolyte replacement or sport drink. A more dilute solution helps limit the number of calories in the drink—a factor that is particularly important for riders who are trying to lose weight. When properly formulated the drink can still maintain optimal hydration and the "drive to drink."

| Fluid Intake Recommendations During Exercise |
|---|
| Two hours prior to exercise, drink 17 to 20 ounces. |
| Every 10 to 20 minutes during exercise, drink 7 to 10 ounces; practically speaking, take a "good gulp"—three to four ounces—every 10 to 15 minutes. |
| After exercise, drink 16 to 24 ounces per pound of body weight lost; practically speaking, minimize body weight loss by adequately hydrating during the ride. |
| Casa, D.J. et al. (2000). National Athletic Trainers' Association: Position statement: Fluid replacement for athletes. Used by permission. |

Table 20-1. Fluid intake recommendations during exercise

*Room temperature.* From either a heat injury or a performance perspective, too cool is always better than a room that is too hot or humid. Even indoors, participants can layer and strip off a long jersey or other light shell after they warm up and the ride is up to speed.

# Taking a Closer Look at Sweat

Why do most people love to sweat? The reasons individuals like to perspire are varied and many. Some are well-founded, but most are based on myths

*Dripping with sweat.* A number of enthusiasts judge the effectiveness of workouts by how much sweat is coursing down their bodies. Excessive sweat accumulation creates the sense of hard work being accomplished and the misguided perception that "if some sweat is good, more must be better." Sweat is not disgusting or improper. It is a natural, rather pure and an inevitable product of exercising. On the other hand, the effectiveness of a workout, in terms of fat loss, calories burned and cardiovascular conditioning, bears little relationship to how much sweat is produced. What counts is the *amount* and *type of activity.*

*The science.* When people exercise, the body produces excess heat as muscles turn fuel into energy. Skin plays a role in keeping the body cool. Blood carries excess heat from deep inside the body to the skin, which allows heat to radiate from the skin's surface. This blood shunt or transfer is exemplified by a red face or flushed skin (due to vasodilation of the blood vessels) on a hot day or in an over-heated classroom.

Meanwhile, the body perspires, dumping water on the skin. The evaporation of sweat cools the body. Through perspiration and breathing, fluid and heat are lost. This fluid comes from blood plasma; profuse sweating reduces blood volume. Blood supply and volume decrease. The blood shunt from the core of the body and decreased blood volume (from sweating and dehydration) cause the heart to beat more times per minute to meet the exercise oxygen needs of working skeletal and heart muscle.

*Practical guidelines for staying cool.* Even a moderate amount of exercise can bring a rider's core temperature up to 100 or 101 degrees (37.5-38 degrees Celsius). Among the steps that can be taken to cool the body include drinking three to four ounces of fluid every 10 to 15 minutes while exercising; wearing loose or "breathable" clothing, which helps the body's cooling system by letting air flow over the skin; and working out in an environment that is well-ventilated and slightly cool upon entering the exercise room.

## Key Point

*The effort by exercisers to attain "dripping-wet" status is counterproductive from a safety, performance and calorie burning standpoint.*

*The perfect temperature.* Research indicates that 55 degrees Fahrenheit (13 degrees Celsius) is the highest temperature at which individuals can expect to perform their best. Temperature is not the sole cause of heat problems. Heat plus humidity (partly influenced by poor ventilation) is more dangerous. Cool and well-ventilated environments present the best conditions for challenging cardiovascular workouts. Do not further increase the temperature and humidity levels by turning up the thermostat, closing off ventilation or wearing an excessive amount of clothing in order to retain heat and sweat more. If the classroom is too cool, participants can add clothing. On the other hand, if rooms are overheated, individuals are more compromised with regard to clothing and hydration options.

*Sweating for weight loss.* Excessively hot environments and layered clothing can promote a loss in body weight via sweating/water loss. Individuals who wear plastic and rubberized suits to increase perspiration can dangerously compromise the cooling system. Neither situation allows evaporation and cooling to occur. Exercisers can lose several pounds of water by sweating, as measured by a scale, in one hour or so. It takes considerable time and effort to lose one pound of fat. Because of the deceiving, instantly gratifying "weight-loss" feedback generated by the scale, many participants are encouraged to, or strive to, "sweat off the pounds." The majority of weight lost is water, which will be replaced when exercisers resume normal fluid and food intake.

*Men compared to women.* Gender can also play a significant role in how individuals respond to core temperature increases. Heat is a limiting factor in physical performance. Metabolic heat consists of higher internal body temperature which is generated by physical activity. Ambient heat is related to environmental temperature and interacts with humidity to produce thermal stress on the body. Researchers have found that women have a higher body temperature at rest than men, fewer sweat glands, lower sweat production, tend to start sweating at higher temperatures than men, and a greater amount of adipose tissue serves as insulation, which inhibits heat dissipation. Men, on the other hand, make greater use of evaporative cooling to manage heat. Men and women handle excess heat in different ways. All factors considered—women have less tolerance to heat than men.

*The bottom line on sweating.* The quantity of sweat and onset of sweating is not a valid measure of what constitutes effective exercise. Too many people erroneously believe that "The harder I work, the more I'll sweat." Furthermore, "Those individuals who are not sweating aren't working hard enough." Neither statement is true.

Is it wrong to "drip with sweat?" Of course not! If riders work at an exercise intensity that has been progressively attained; drink lots of fluid before, during and after their workout sessions; wear appropriate clothing that enhances the cooling processes of the body; and are in a cool and well-ventilated environment—they still might end up "dripping wet" with sweat.

## Key Point

*Training without proper fluid intake does not "toughen" anyone. Doing so simply makes individuals better at training when they are dehydrated—a point at which they are nowhere near top performance capabilities.*

# Fueling Workouts

When and what riders eat can dramatically affect performance and recovery. The timing and types of nutrients to ingest are well-documented. Coaches can help guide students in making sound nutritional choices before, during and after the ryde.

*What riders should eat.* If participants work out three to five times per week at moderate-to-hard levels of effort—and optimal performance is not one of the training goals—glycogen stores can be replenished with a regular diet that is high in carbohydrate (60 to 65 percent of daily calorie intake).

*Serious riding.* Riders who work out twice a day and race regularly should pay close attention to recovery diet. Individuals often fail to follow a proper recovery diet because they are unaware of its importance to next-day training or long-term performance.

Within 15 minutes after exercise has stopped, begin to replace any fluid losses with juices, foods high in water (the kind that run down the face when eaten), sport drinks and water.

If the rider waits longer to feed, glycogen stores will not be replenished as quickly. About 300 calories are needed within two hours of finishing the ride. Carbohydrate rich foods and beverages are the proper food choice for recovery. This initial feeding should be followed with about 300 additional carbohydrate calories every two hours thereafter, for six to eight hours. In total, this schedule entails three to four 300-calorie carbohydrate feedings over six to eight hours. Combine protein with carbohydrate-recovery foods. Protein, like carbohydrate, stimulates the production of insulin, which helps "herd" blood glucose into the muscles to enhance glycogen replacement.

**Key Point**

*Nutritional priorities for all cyclists who train regularly include carbohydrate, protein and electrolyte/fluid replenishment before, during and after the ryde.*

# 21

# Apparel and Footwear Guidelines

This story is timeless. Kids of parents who cycle always have, and will continue to ridicule cycling attire. A basic ugliness and garish nature of the typical costume worn by cyclists is undeniable. In time, as the kids of cyclists begin to ride, their laughter and ridicule sheepishly transforms and simply ends with, "Can you get me a pair of those?" Function over-rules cool!

**Key Point**

*It has been said: "If you are going to ride a bike, you should look like you are riding a bike!"*

Common sense always comes to the forefront when butts hurt, legs are chaffed and there is nowhere to store a tube or food. Proper apparel, protective gear and cycling shoes have a positive impact on the entire riding experience.

*Gear.* The short and long of what—and what not to use—is very straightforward. Do not wear cotton; do use a towel indoors; keep laces tucked into the shoes; purchase cycling shorts; ride with a synthetic jersey; consider riding with a cap and/or wear a headband or skull bandana to keep sweat out of the eyes. Cycling gloves are not needed indoors—they are good for grip and padding—but stink like nasty socks if they are not washed regularly.

Riding apparel, cycling shoes and assorted gear contribute to:

- Function
- Comfort
- Safety
- Performance enhancement, enjoyment and compliance

## Apparel and Riding Gear Considerations:

- Magnify cooling effects by wearing synthetic jerseys; they dry quickly and wick moisture.
- Wear padded cycling shorts with a chamois in order to increase comfort and limit abrasive contact and pressure points between the saddle and the inner thighs, including several high stress points in the buttocks area (pubis symphysis and ischial tuberosities).
- Avoid baggy or extremely loose-fitting cotton clothing.
- Use bandanas, headbands, towels or light cotton bike caps to absorb sweat.
- Launder cycling garments (jerseys, shirts, cycling shorts, socks) and any other washable gear after each workout; abrasion/friction and sweat create a spawning ground for skin infection.
- Consider using saddle covers (e.g., gel) to disperse pressure; gel seats are especially helpful to novice riders or individuals who ride once or twice per week.
- Use specially designed (anatomically correct) saddles; ergonomically designed seats are available for both female and male anatomy; designs accommodate larger hip widths and anatomical/gender-specific pressure points.

# Footwear Guidelines

The RealRyder bike comes with two-sided pedals. SPD (Shimano Pedaling Dynamics), or clipless pedals are on one side and conventional toe clips on the flip-side accommodate any athletic tennis-type shoe. Clipless cycling shoes are highly recommended. For first-time riders, "clipping into the pedal" with a "clipless" shoe is not essential. As riding skills improve and the rider wants to achieve a better pedal stroke, the use of clipless pedals becomes increasingly important. The shoe/pedal link attaches the rider to the bike and greatly impacts pedal stroke mechanics. In addition, cycling shoes feature stiffer soles—which maximize power transfer and efficiency.

*Clipless pedal history.* Clipless pedals (as well as clip-in or step-in) require a special cycling shoe that has a cleat fitted to the sole—which locks into a mechanism in the pedal that holds the shoe firmly to the pedal. Most *clipless* pedals currently available on the market lock to the cleats when stepped into firmly and unlock when the foot is twisted outward. The term *clipless* refers to the lack of an external toe clip (cage). The clipless pedal was invented by Charles Hanson in 1895. It allowed the rider to twist the shoe to lock and unlock, and had rotational float (the freedom to rotate the shoe slightly to prevent foot/knee strain).

In 1971, Cino Cinelli designed a more advanced clipless pedal, the M71. Cinelli's pedal employed a plastic shoe cleat, which slid into grooves in the pedal and locked in place, with a small lever located on the back side of the pedal body. To release the shoe, a rider had to reach down and operate the lever, similar to the way a racing cyclist had to reach down and loosen the toestrap of a cage (toe clip). Because of the need to reach down to the lever to unclip the pedal, Cinelli's pedals have often been referred to as "death cleats."

In 1984, the French company LOOK borrowed from downhill snow ski binding technology and produced the first widely used *clipless* pedals. The next major development in clipless pedals was Shimano's SPD (Shimano Pedaling Dynamics) pedal system. SPD cleats are small and can be fitted into a recess in the sole, making it possible to walk more easily when off the bike—a feature that is particularly useful when mountain biking or riding indoors.

*Clipless shoes.* Combined with a stiff-soled shoe, the clipless system employed on a RealRyder bike—stepping into and attaching the foot via an SPD pedal—offers great energy savings. All of the energy that a rider's leg and foot bring to the pedal goes to the pedal. Because the shoe is clipped into the pedal, as the foot goes through the revolution of the crank, participants can pedal more efficiently through the entire pedal stroke.

*The toe clip/cage.* A toe clip set-up allows the foot to bend. Some energy is lost when the power of the leg and foot is transferred to the pedal. Toe clips, on the other hand, can be used with any shoe, and require little or no maintenance. Getting into the toe-clip system can be challenging because the rider must flip the pedal up and strap in. The straps cause the pedal to hang upside-down when not in use. With practice, this technique becomes easier, but it is never as easy or efficient compared to clipless pedals.

*Shoe maintenance.* Shoes can be sprayed or rubbed with a conditioner. The toe-clip system requires almost no maintenance. Clipless pedals and the cleat on each shoe should be lubricated more often, especially if the participants ride in wet and muddy conditions, or in the case of riding indoors, they sweat a lot. If the cleat starts to feel like it is getting "sticky" or is not clicking into or out of the pedal smoothly, it is time for cleaning and lubricant.

*Changing out pedals.* Serious riders may want to bring in their own pedals and swap them out for the ride. Each facility generally sets policy regarding this option. Riders must know how to properly loosen and thread pedals onto the crank arm. Improper pedal removal or attachment can cause damage to the crank arms or create safety concerns for the next rider. Participants should be encouraged to purchase SPD compatible cleats and cycling shoes—and clip in for a RealRyde.

# Appendix A: Incorporating Authentic Cycling Language

Instructors who bring years of road cycling experience into the classroom, or take time to "speak the language," can energize any indoor cycling experience. Cycling stands heavily on its jargon, nomenclature and history. An entire ride can be created based on the lingo of the sport.

**Key Point**

*Cycling language can be used to create individual challenges and monotony-breaking imagery.*

*How language works.* Let's roll...In a "breakaway" some riders are asked to lead the pack—the breakaway group. This road race strategy allows the breakaway group to push effort, while the rest of the group (peloton) recovers in the "draft" created by the pack of riders (peloton) that they are "hanging in" on. On cue, the peloton can be encouraged to "go with," "bring back," or "chase" the breakaway group.

Using RydingSlang contributes to limitless creativity. The energy cycling language brings to a class in terms of anticipation and fun is significant. The variety it can usher into the classroom can relieve the "same-old" aspect that can infect indoor cycling classes over time.

**Key Point**

*Cyclists do not always want to focus on gears, riding form and drills. Sometimes, they "just want to ride" and match what the environment and opponent throws at them.*

## RydingSlang

A myriad of language options exist that help create a ride that requires responses and emotions to the scenario that is set up by the use of colorful, engaging language:

- *"Breakaway, sprint, jumping on it, jump, attack"* refers to a situation where a single or a group of riders display a burst of speed.
- *"Chase"* refers to riding hard to catch a breakaway group.

- *"Drafting"* or *"riding the slipstream"* refers to riding in a lead cyclist's slipstream, which can save as much as 30% of the effort by avoiding wind resistance.
- *"To pull"* refers to leading the pack (peloton) or pace-line of riders; the "animal" with the "guns" (strong legs; oversized quads) often "leads out" and "pulls."
- *"Pull off"* refers to peeling from the lead and taking a drafting position at the end of the pace-line, pack or field of riders; this action allows all riders in the pace-line to ride hard, pushes the overall effort and mph by establishing strong "leads," and builds in recovery so that the performance level/speed of the riders can be sustained.
- *"Pull through"* refers to the second rider in a pace-line and the point at which that participant takes over the front position; the previous leader, who is done "pulling," pulls off and takes a position at the back of the pace-line.
- *"Hanging on"* or *"sitting in"* refers to a rider who constantly "drafts" and never "pulls" or takes a turn leading the pack. This situation is considered contemptuous, unless of course, the rider has permission of the group to do so, and the group has agreed to "carry" that person.
- *"Reeling-in"* refers to the chase group of riders regaining contact with the breakaway group; this usually requires a larger group that is working in a "pace-line" that can sustain a higher speed than a small breakaway group, making it very hard for the small breakaway group to make the attempt "stick."
- *"Shifting up"* refers to increasing intensity (e.g., the size of gear or the amount of resistance).
- *"Shifting down"* refers to decreasing intensity (e.g., the size of gear or the amount of resistance).
- *"Pick up a gear, click up a gear, lose a gear, click down a gear, add a gear, drop a gear, click up two"* refers to an appropriate transition from flats to hill climb or vice versa, so that the rider has the right amount of "gear" or resistance (increasing or decreasing).
- *"Forcing the pace"* refers to increasing the speed of the ride to the point where other riders are having trouble keeping up, which puts those riders into "difficulty."
- *"Suffering"* requires no explanation. You are pushing very hard or can no longer keep the pace.
- *"Difficulty"* refers to a situation in which the demands of the ride are somewhat overwhelming to a participant; riders are said to be "placed into difficulty" when an opponent or terrain present a challenge that results in them "falling off the pace" and entering into a huge degree of personal "suffering" or "difficulty."
- *"Hammering"* refers to riding hard seated or standing.
- *"Field sprint"* refers to a sprint for the finish line that involves a large pack of riders; this burst of speed entails an all out sprint.
- *"Free-ride home"* refers to a situation when the ride is over; riders are cooling down; everyone is returning "home," using any technique or style of riding they choose.

- *"Taking the wind, getting into the wind, on the front"* refers to a teammate who "takes the wind" for a rider, as the team leader does not want to waste energy on the front; if the rider is a "domestique" and sacrifices himself for teammates, that individual will be taking a lot of wind out on the front of the "pace line" or "peloton."
- *"Drafting, getting on a wheel, finding a wheel"* refers to participants getting behind another rider and letting that person break the wind for them, which allows them to use much less energy.
- *"Sitting in"* refers to drafting on a group of riders and not doing any attacking or undertaking a fair share of work "on the front." Riders may be "sitting in" to save themselves for the end of the race or, they may be "sitting in" because they are exhausted and want to "finish the ride." If capable, etiquette says that all riders share the front position on the peloton or in a breakaway group.
- *"Rolling or rolling in"* refers to a situation that is similar to the previous definition of "sitting in;" in this instance, the riders are tired. They are just going to "roll" or cruise to the finish.
- *"Peloton or main group"* refers to the mass of riders in a race; as they split apart more than one peloton can exist in the same ride.
- *"Echelon"* refers to a group of riders taking their "turn" on the front blocking the wind. An echelon will constantly rotate, and a "turn" typically will last only a few seconds. This technique is a group-riding skill that every racer needs to master. As a rule, an echelon is undertaken in two lines, with one line going up and the other line back. The scenario can be created indoors.
- *"Rotating"* refers to a period of time in which riders take their "turn" at the front of a group, a break or their turn in a quickly moving echelon.
- *"Attacking"* refers to an increase of speed and power that is designed to enable riders to "gap" or "separate" from their opponents. A key to attacking is to do so at a point that the competition would rather not work hard or can no longer match the effort. A single rider can "attack" in order to create a "solo break."
- *"Sort out the group"* refers to riders forcing the pace to find out who can match the attack. This results in the group splitting with the weaker riders left behind.
- *"Get in the wind"* refers to a situation when individuals "sort out the group"; riders are forced to "get in the wind" to match the attacking effort. By their actions, they are asking, "Who is going with me, and who isn't?"
- *"Suck air and hammer the legs"* refers to a strategy wherein, if another team's top rider is a strong sprinter, participants might want to attack into a hill at a fast, punishing race pace. That way, the sprinter will become fatigued, and hopefully "suck air and hammer the legs," with the end result being less energy for a final sprint attempt. Likely, that rider will have nothing left (running on empty) and will fail or "bonk" in the sprint attempt.
- *"Drop or dropped"* refers to a situation when participants cannot ride as hard as the rest of the riders, and they fall off race-pace, with no hope of "catching back on" or "coming back into contact" with the group.

- *"Catching back on"* refers to a situation that occurs when participants get dropped and then "ride back to the group"; having to "ride back" is a huge waste of energy; the key is to avoid being "dropped."
- *"Gap"* refers to spaces between riders, which greatly influences whether individuals can take advantage of a draft; riders like to "close the gap."
- *"Bridging"* refers to riding across a "gap" from one group to another, which usually requires an acceleration.
- *"Blocking"* refers to purposely riding slowly on the front, after a rider has attacked.
- *"A break,"* whether solo or a group, refers to an attack that is trying to "stay away" from the main group until the ride/race is finished.
- *"Reeling in a break"* or *"catching a break"* and *"covering a break/attack"* refers to a situation where riders are working hard to neutralize an attack that turned into a "break" that separated riders.
- *"Counter or counterattack"* refers to attacking immediately after a separate attack has been neutralized. Attacking and then counterattacking a team over and over can have a devastating physical and mental impact.
- *"Putting the head down," "time trialing,"* or *"TT"* refers to riding full out, with no focus other than riding hard, efficient and with a big power/speed output. If riders initiate a solo break, they "put their head down" and "go." If they get dropped on a hill, they get to the top, "put their head down," and try to "catch back on."
- *"Using a match"* or *"using the last stick"* refers to a hypothetical situation in which riders believe that in any race, each rider has a box of wood-stick matches. More talented riders have a larger "box of sticks." Individuals can only attack so many times, or cover a break so many times. Each effort that pushes them out of their comfort zone costs them a "stick." While it is great to use a match or a stick, the trick is to never run out. On the other hand, no one wants to finish with too many sticks left in the box—especially if they are racing. An example of an on the bike commentary from teammate to teammate might sound like, "So, how many matches do you have left? Are you all burned up? No, sticks left? Whatchugot?" Riders will test one another to burn up "sticks" and to gauge how "deep" each rider can go into the "pain cave."

# Rolling In

The only limitation to using traditional cycling language is one's comfort level using the language. Individuals who watch any classic cycling race, by the end of the race, can use the same language as the race commentators with ease. Using rider-in-the-know slang will enhance any indoor riding experience.

All participants will enjoy an infusion of cycling language and the imagery it paints. They will also benefit from the competitive riding scenarios that are created. Using cycling language during RealRyder indoor class rides—brings the fun.

# Appendix B:
# RealRyder Pilot Study

**Loy, Steven et al., 2009, Cal State University—Northridge (CSUN)**

## Study Highlights

The objective of this investigation was to determine the energy cost and muscle involvement during specific activities performed on a RealRyder cycle in a 1) locked stationary or 2) an unlocked RealRyder cycle set-up—which allows for natural side-to-side bike movement. The primary intent of the comparison between the sit/lock and sit/unlock and the comparable stand/lock and stand/unlock positions was to identify any changes in $VO_2$ (energy cost/calorie expenditure) that occurred with a "stable" ride versus the "free" RealRyder cycle ride. The study also looked at muscle activation, with special focus on the positions where the RealRyder cycle is turned, banked or ridden with a lean.

Several key differences were found, including:

❑ When comparing the RealRyder cycle in the locked (stationary) vs. an unlocked (unstationary) position, while *standing (not turning)*…

- The results confirm that both the $O_2$ uptake (calories utilized) and heart rate (HR) increase by about 10 percent, using the "unlocked" RealRyder cycle.

❑ The most dramatic caloric and HR differences between a traditional stationary indoor cycle and the RealRyder indoor cycle exist while *standing and turning*…

- The results confirm a 25% increase in the number of calories utilized (2.2-2.3/min) and a 20 percent increase in heart rate.

Dr. Loy and his colleagues reported that "In the standing position, the greatest values were obtained during the turns, followed by the unlocked condition, followed by the locked condition." The RealRyder utilizes more calories when compared to a fixed stationary bike "when turning," whether seated or standing.

❑ It is interesting to note that on a road bike, energy costs also increase about 10 percent when moving from a seated to a standing position. The articulating RealRyder cycle compares favorably to the energy costs of a road bike, because it provides a "real" ride.

The following data details the increase in $VO_2$/oxygen consumption that occurs when moving from a seated to a standing position on both a fixed stationary set-up and a RealRyder cycle:

| Fixed stationary bike set-up: | RealRyder cycle: |
|---|---|
| Seated, locked = 33.37 $O_2$ (ml/kg/min) | Seated, unlocked = 33.37 $O_2$ (ml/kg/min) |
| Standing, locked = 34.46 $O_2$ | Standing, unlocked= 37.18 $O_2$ |
| —3.0 percent increase | —11.4 percent increase |

*Oblique activation.* The activation and strengthening of the obliques while riding (steering, leaning and turning) the RealRdyer cycle is an exceptional feature that increases core stability in both pro and novice riders. In addition to what occurs in a seated position while riding straight, oblique activation is increased even more significantly when turning the RealRyder cycle.

The results of the pilot study have been incorporated into the programming efforts of RealRyder to help riders be more successful and effective. These study results provide insight that help instructors teach more effectively.

# The RealRyder Cycle Pilot Study: An Overview

The objective of this study was to determine the energy cost and muscle involvement during specific activities on the RealRyder cycle. The investigation examined the difference between a locked (stationary) and normal, and an unlocked RealRyder cycle set-up, which allows for natural bike movement under the rider. The primary intent of the comparison between the sit/lock and sit/unlock and the comparable stand/lock and stand/unlock was to identify any changes in $VO_2$ (energy cost/calorie expenditure) that occurred with a "stable" ride versus the "free" RealRyder cycle ride. The study also looked at muscle activation levels, especially in the positions where the RealRyder cycle is turned, banked or ridden with a lean.

❑ *Seated and standing with lean.* Riding the RealRyder cycle, with a lean in both seated and standing positions, resulted in an increased caloric cost of ~2 kcal/min. When extrapolated over the course of a 30-minute ride that change equates to an additional 60 kcal/min, which projects out to an additional pound of weight loss in two months of daily riding. The turning protocol was not unrealistic, given the return to center between every turn for about 10 seconds. From this limited sample size, it would appear that the relative increase in oxygen consumption is similar, whether sitting or standing, but differences may exist at higher levels of intensities (cadence or load increases) of exercise, which may require different muscle recruitment.

❑ *Seated and standing—locked vs. unlocked.* In this area, the study's findings presented a surprise to both the researchers and the RealRyder team. The accepted hypothesis of everyone involved was that seated or standing *unlocked* (free movement under the rider) riding would equate to greater caloric expenditure, when compared to seated or standing *locked* riding for a given cadence and work load (resistance). That situation, however, did not occur. The key to this puzzling situation is to first remember that every subject emphasized how much they preferred the free-ride (unlocked) position, compared to the fixed (locked) position. More or less, it was reported that the ride in an unlocked position felt easier, smoother and more natural. In other words, fixed stationary cycles are more costly to ride in terms of stress. It is more efficient to ride a freely moving bike that is properly designed. It should be noted that many stationary bikes fail at the bottom bracket, since the mechanical stress that exists at that point cannot be dissipated effectively, without a natural movement/lean occurring when riding. This factor, of course, happens on both a road cycle and the RealRyder cycle, because of the articulating bike frame.

❏ *Discussion.* An issue arises concerning why the heart rate (HR) and $VO_2$ decrease in the aforementioned comparison. It is hypothesized that the drop in HR and $VO_2$ is because of the "functional efficiency" of riding "unlocked" versus "locked." Anecdotally, it has been observed that it is easier to work harder and longer on the RealRyder cycle than it is on a fixed stationary bike. Research which found that the "fatigue threshold" is most influenced by local muscle fatigue, rather than by the limits of the heart and lungs, supports this conclusion. An explanation of the functional efficiency of the "free" (naturally articulating) RealRyder bike frame design, at both the low-end of effort (seated, riding straight) and the high-end of effort (emptying the tank), is addressed in detail in the RealRyder instructor training program.

# The Design and Set-Up of the Pilot Study

The study examined the following activity-specific variables:

❏ *Sitting or standing while riding:*

- With the RealRyder cycle in a "locked" position
- With the RealRyder cycle in an "unlocked," normal RealRyder cycle position
- With the RealRyder cycle in an "unlocked," normal RealRyder cycle position; the turning adhered to a protocol of three seconds to shift to a full-right turn and holding the turn for seven seconds, followed by a return to center in three seconds, and then holding center for seven seconds, followed by a three-second shift to a full-left turn, and then holding the turn for seven seconds. This protocol was repeated until steady state metabolism was achieved.
- After the locked ride, the stabilizing blocks were removed to achieve a normal RealRyder cycle position, which allows for natural bike movement under the rider.

Table B-1 provides a statistical overview of the study, which looked at how the variables were affected with regard to the following four factors:

- Max $VO_2$ (ml/kg/min)
- Caloric cost (kcal/min)
- Heart rate (bpm)
- Respiratory quotient (rq)

| Max VO$_2$ (ml/kg/min) | 49.7 | 49.4 | 48.1 | 65.0 | 81.1 | 58.7 | | |
|---|---|---|---|---|---|---|---|---|
| **Relative O$_2$ (ml/kg/min)** | Sub 1 | Sub 2 | Sub 3 | Sub 4 | Sub 5 | Avg. | St. Dev. | Avg % VO$_2$ max |
| Sit/Lock | 25.40 | 24.95 | 29.40 | 39.05 | 48.05 | 33.37 | 9.97 | 56.4 |
| Sit/Unlock | 23.10 | 24.8 | 24.60 | 37.10 | 43.20 | 30.56 | 9.04 | 51.7 |
| Sit/Turns | 31.20 | 32.3 | 32.25 | 41.10 | 48.40 | 37.05** | 7.50 | 63.6 |
| Stand/Lock | 28.80 | 29.9 | 25.50 | 41.10 | 47.00 | 34.46 | 9.14 | 58.5 |
| Stand/Unlock | 30.00 | 35.3 | 28.10 | 43.50 | 49.00 | 37.18 | 8.90 | 63.4 |
| Stand/Turns | 38.80 | 38.5 | 37.30 | 48.00 | 55.20 | 43.56** | 7.79 | 75.1 |
| **Caloric Cost (Kcal/min)** | Sub 1 | Sub 2 | Sub 3 | Sub 4 | Sub 5 | Avg. | St. Dev. | |
| Sit/Lock | 7.80 | 7.30 | 11.90 | 14.05 | 15.15 | 11.24 | 3.57 | |
| Sit/Unlock | 7.10 | 7.25 | 9.90 | 13.30 | 13.60 | 10.23 | 3.15 | |
| Sit/Turns | 9.65 | 9.50 | 13.05 | 14.75 | 15.25 | 12.44** | 2.74 | |
| Stand/Lock | 8.80 | 8.7 | 8.50 | 14.80 | 14.80 | 11.12 | 3.36 | |
| Stand/Unlock | 9.20 | 10.4 | 11.40 | 15.70 | 15.50 | 12.44 | 2.99 | |
| Stand/Turns | 12.20 | 11.5 | 15.20 | 17.50 | 17.60 | 14.80** | 2.87 | |
| **Heart-Rate (Beats/min)** | Sub 1 | Sub 2 | Sub 3 | Sub 4 | Sub 5 | Avg. | St. Dev. | |
| Sit/Lock | 140 | 146 | 131 | 140 | 149 | 141.2 | 6.91 | |
| Sit/Unlock | 134 | 145 | 128 | 137 | 145 | 137.8 | 7.33 | |
| Sit/Turns | 164 | 171 | 141 | 146 | 159 | 156.2** | 12.48 | |
| Stand/Lock | 162 | 165 | 145 | 150 | 158 | 156.0 | 8.34 | |
| Stand/Unlock | 164 | 180 | 150 | 158 | 164 | 163.2 | 11.01 | |
| Stand/Turns | 185 | 193 | 165 | 165 | 175 | 176.6** | 12.36 | |
| **Respiratory Quotient (RQ)** | Sub 1 | Sub 2 | Sub 3 | Sub 4 | Sub 5 | Avg. | St. Dev. | |
| Sit/Lock | 0.92 | 0.93 | 0.97 | 0.91 | 0.92 | 0.93 | 0.03 | |
| Sit/Unlock | 0.90 | 0.90 | 0.95 | 0.90 | 0.92 | 0.91 | 0.02 | |
| Sit/Turns | 0.94 | 0.93 | 0.95 | 0.91 | 0.92 | 0.93 | 0.02 | |
| Stand/Lock | 0.89 | 0.88 | 1.00 | 0.94 | 0.92 | 0.93 | 0.05 | |
| Stand/Unlock | 0.90 | 0.94 | 0.97 | 0.94 | 0.94 | 0.94 | 0.02 | |
| Stand/Turns | 1.08 | 1.01 | 1.00 | 0.98 | 0.97 | 1.01 | 0.04 | |

** Turns greater than the unlocked position ($P < 0.05$).

Table B-1. Results of the RealRyder pilot study

The percent $VO_2$max of the seated rides would be considered of moderate intensity. Riders were allowed to self-select a cadence, and the resistance was adjusted to be between 50 and 60 percent $VO_2$max. With the resistance adjustment, it is very challenging to achieve a specific $VO_2$ value.

The percent $VO_2$max for the standing rides was achieved by first having subjects stand and select a cadence at which they were comfortable and could be maintained with a resistance that permitted a similar percent $VO_2$max that they attained in the sit/lock position. All factors considered, the researcher team was reasonably successful at obtaining the targeted intensity of exercise.

The primary intent of the comparison between the sit/lock and sit/unlock and the comparable stand/lock and stand/unlock was to identify any changes in $VO_2$ that occurred with a "stable" ride versus the "free" RealRyder ride.

# Center and Turning Positions

❏ *Turning.* A key issue that the study attempted to examine was a comparison of the center position to the turning position in both the sitting and standing positions. In fact, an appropriate comparison can be made between the center position and the turning position, while both sitting and standing, since the resistance was not altered in either. The differences that were found are striking.

In the sitting position, all subjects evidenced an increase on each of the four factors, with averages of:

- +11.9 percent $VO_2$max
- +2.2 kcal/min
- +18.4 bpm
- +0.02 RQ, reflecting an estimated 6.6 percent increase in carbohydrate requirement for the activity

In the standing position, all subjects evidenced an increase with averages of:

- +11.7 percent $VO_2$max
- +2.36 kcal/min
- +13.4 bpm
- +0.7 RQ, reflecting an estimated 19.3 percent increase in carbohydrate requirement in the activity, though it is suggested that this increase is *not* indicative of the activity alone but also reflects an increase in $CO_2$ production related to lactate production, since the exercise intensity was rather high for the lesser-conditioned subjects.

As demonstrated, the increased caloric cost of ~2 kcal/min, when extrapolated over the course of a 30-minute ride, is 60 kcal/min. Projected, this factor could result in an additional pound of weight loss in two months of daily riding. The turning protocol was not unrealistic, given the return to center between every turn for about 10 seconds. The aforementioned results above could be magnified. From this limited sample size, it seems that the relative increase in oxygen consumption is similar, whether sitting or standing, with turning. On the other hand, differences at higher intensities of exercise may exist that might require different muscle recruitment.

# EMG

Six muscles were examined for a three-second interval during each condition (locked, unlocked, left turn, right turn) for each position (seated, standing). Two of the muscles that were investigated were "core" muscles—erector spinae and external oblique. The other four were upper-extremity muscles—biceps, triceps, traps and middle deltoid. Because electrodes were placed on only one side of the body, the results illustrated in Figures B-1 and B-2 should be interpreted with this factor in mind, particularly when evaluating the turning data. Researchers made the assumption that electrodes on the other side of the body would have produced similar results. Each sample was collected at the approximate midpoint in time of the condition protocol. During the turns, the three-second interval was collected when the rider was at the maximum deviation from the central position. Each muscle was expressed as a percentage of the maximum voluntary isometric contraction.

As can be seen by examining the standard deviation bars on Figures B-1 and B-2, muscle-activation responses were highly variable. For statistical purposes, bilateral symmetry was assumed for all positions/conditions. Therefore, the right and left sides were summed for the turns and doubled for the two straight-ahead conditions.

# Statistics

Because of the small sample size, normal distribution was not assumed, and nonparametric tests were used. To determine if differences existed between conditions, a Friedman two-way ANOVA was conducted. If statistical significance was found, Wilcoxon matched tests were used, post-hoc, to determine which conditions were different.

# Results

The same trends were observed for relative $O_2$, caloric cost and heart rate. In the seated position, the greatest values were obtained during the turns, followed by the locked condition, followed by the unlocked condition. In the standing position, the greatest values were obtained during the turns, followed by the unlocked condition, followed by the locked condition. RQ was not significantly different between conditions for either position.

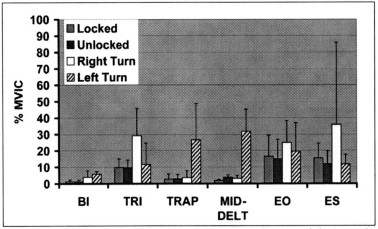

Figure B-1. Muscle activation in the various conditions, while seated

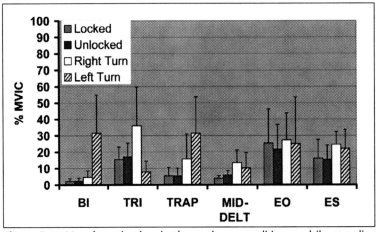

Figure B-2. Muscle activation in the various conditions, while standing

EMG activity was not significantly different between the locked and unlocked conditions. Certain muscles, however, exhibited greater activity during the turns. In both the seated and standing position, the biceps, traps, and middle deltoids all had greater activation during the turns. In addition, in the seated position, the triceps and external obliques had greater contributions. In neither position did the erector spinae exhibit increased activation. Increased muscle activation, particularly of the upper body, may explain (in part) the increased oxygen consumption during the turns. Such a hypothesis, however, requires further testing. Specifically, a larger number of subjects would need to be tested, the resistance on the wheel would need to be quantified, and a larger number of muscles would need to be examined.

# References and Suggested Reading

American College of Sports Medicine (ACSM). (2009). *ACSM Guidelines For Exercise Testing and Prescription,* 8th edition. Philadelphia, PA: Wolters Kluwer/Lippincott Williams & Wilkins

Anthony, Lenita (1996). Getting in Gear. *IDEA Personal Trainer.* July/August

Anthony, Lenita (1996). Bringing Cycling Indoors. *IDEA Today.* June

Asker, E. Jeukendrup (2002). *High-Performance Cycling.* Champaign, IL: Human Kinetics

Barry, D., Barry, M., and Sovndal, S. (2006). *Fitness Cycling,* 2nd ed. Champaign, IL: Human Kinetics

Brooks, Douglas (2004). *The Complete Book of Personal Training.* Champaign, IL: Human Kinetics

Burke, E.R. (2003). *High-Tech Cycling,* 2nd ed. Champaign, IL: Human Kinetics

Burke, E.R. (2002). *Serious Cycling*, 2nd ed. Champaign, IL: Human Kinetics

Caldwell, G.E., et al. (1999). Lower-extremity joint moments during uphill cycling. *Journal of Applied Biomechanics,* 15, 2, 166-181

Casa, D.J. et al. (2000). National Athletic Trainers' Association: Position statement: Fluid replacement for athletes. *Journal of Athletic Training,* 35, 212-224

Coyle, E.F., et al. (1992). Cycling efficiency is related to the percentage of type I muscle fibers. *Medicine & Science in Sports & Exercise,* 24, 782-788

Dallam, G.M., and Jonas. S. (2008). *Championship Triathlon Training.* Champaign, IL: Human Kinetics

Dishman, R.K., Farquhar, R.P., & Cureton, K.J. (1994). Responses to preferred intensities of exertion in men differing in activity levels. *Medicine and Science in Sports and Exercise* 26 (9): 783-90

Elliot, B., Gaetz, M., & Anderson, G.S. (2004). EMG activity of trunk stabilizers during stable and unstable exercise. *Canadian Journal of Applied Physiology.* 29(supplement):S43(Abstract)

Evans, Marc (2003). *Triathlete's Edge—Advanced training for performance.* Champaign, IL: Human Kinetics

Finch, Michael (2004). *Triathlon Training.* Champaign, IL: Human Kinetics

Hamley, E. & Thomas, V. (1967). Physiological and postural factors in the calibration of a bicycle ergometer. *Journal of Physiology,* 191, 55-57

Hodges, P.W. & Richardson, C.A. (1996) Inefficient muscular stabilization of the lumbar spine associated with LBP: A motor control evaluation of the TVA. *Spine,* 21, 2640-2650.

Holmes, J., Pruitt, A., & Whalen, A. (1994). Lower-extremity overuse in bicycling. In *Clinics in sports medicine,* 13, 1. *Bicycle injuries: Prevention and management,* edited by M.R. Mellion & E.R. Burke, 187-206. Philadelphia: Saunders

Loy, Steven et al. (2009). *RealRyder Cycle Pilot Study.* Cal State University-Northridge (Pilot Study)

Nordeen, K. & Cavanagh, P. (1975). Simulation of lower-limb kinematics during cycling. In *Biomechanics V-B,* edited by P. Komi, 26-33. Baltimore: University Park Press

McCary, Patrick (1986). *The Road to Kona Never Ends.* Greeley, CO: Sports Psychology Publications, Pioneer Press

Mora, John (2009). *Triathlon 101,* 2nd ed. Champaign, IL: Human Kinetics

Plant, Mike (1987). *Iron Will—The Heart and Soul of the Triathlon's Ultimate Challenge.* Chicago, IL: Contemporary Books, Inc.

Post, William R. (1998). Patellofemoral pain, *Physician and SportsMedicine,* Volume 26, No. 1, pp. 68-78, January

Shennum, P. & DeVries, H. (1975). The effect of saddle height on oxygen consumption during bicycle ergometer work. *Medicine & Science in Sports & Exercise,* 8, 199–121

Sovndal, Shannon (2009). *Cycling Anatomy.* Champaign, IL: Human Kinetics

Willardson, J.M. (2007) Core stability training: Applications to sports conditioning programs. *Journal of Strength and Conditioning Research,* 21, 3, 979–985